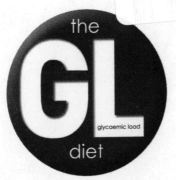

the
# GL
glycaemic load
diet

# NIGEL DENBY

WITH TINA VAN DER HEIJDEN
AND DEBORAH PYNER

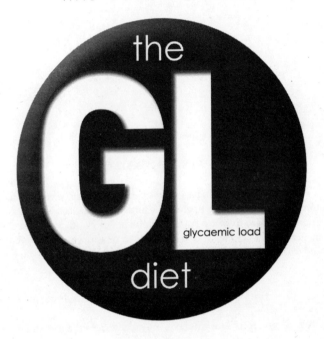

the
**GL**
glycaemic load
diet

JOHN BLAKE

Published by John Blake Publishing Ltd,
3, Bramber Court, 2 Bramber Road,
London W14 9PB, England

www.blake.co.uk

First published in paperback in 2005

ISBN 1 84454 112 6

British Library Cataloguing-in-Publication Data:

A catalogue record for this book is available from the British Library.

Design by www.envydesign.co.uk

Printed in Great Britain by Bookmarque, Croydon

7 9 10 8 6

© Text copyright Nigel Denby, Tina van der Heijden
and Deborah Pyner

Papers used by John Blake Publishing are natural, recyclable
products made from wood grown in sustainable forests.
The manufacturing processes conform to the environmental
regulations of the country of origin.

# Acknowledgements

With many thanks to: Dr Walter Willett – for pioneering the GL diet; Dr Wright – a very busy GP and inspiring gentleman; Michelle and all at John Blake Publishing for all their hard work; long-suffering fabulous friends, partners and families – for being great testers and guinea pigs; all the delightful Diet Freedomers to date who have supported and believed in us and, having lost weight, are now spreading the word.

This publication is meant to be used as a general reference and recipe book to aid weight loss. As with any weight-loss plan, before commencing we would strongly recommend that you consult your doctor to see whether it is a suitable weight-loss plan for you.

The publishers, authors, or Diet Freedom Limited, directly or indirectly, do not dispense medical advice.

While all reasonable care has been taken during the preparation of this book, the publishers, editors or authors cannot accept responsibility for any consequences arising from the use of this information.

This book includes references to nuts and recipes including nuts, nut derivatives and nut oils. Avoid if you have a known allergic reaction. Pregnant and nursing mothers, invalids, the elderly, children and babies may be potentially vulnerable to nut allergies and should therefore avoid nuts, nut derivatives and nut oils.

## A Note on Recipe Conversions

25g = 1 oz
30ml = 1 fl oz

# Contents

# About the Author

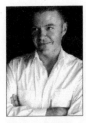 Nigel Denby trained as a dietitian at Glasgow Caledonian University, following an established career in the catering industry. He is also a qualified chef and previously owned his own restaurant.

His dietetic career began as a Research Dietitian at the Human Nutrition Research Centre in Newcastle upon Tyne. After a period working as a Community Dietitian, Nigel left the NHS to join Boots Health and Beauty Experience, where he led the delivery and training of Nutrition and Weight Management services.

In 2003, Nigel set up his own nutrition consultancy, delivering a clinical service to Hammersmith and Queen Charlotte's Hospital Women's Health Clinic and the International Eating Disorders Centre in Buckinghamshire as well as acting as Nutrition Consultant for the Childbase Children's Nursery Group.

Nigel also runs his own private practice in Harley Street,

specialising in weight management, PMS/ menopause, irritable bowel syndrome and food intolerance.

Nigel works extensively with the media, writing for the *Sunday Telegraph Magazine*, *Zest*, *Essentials* and various other consumer magazines. His work in radio and television includes BBC and ITN news programmes, Channel 4's *Fit Farm*, BBC Breakfast and BBC *Real Story*.

# Introduction

I remember the very first time I went on a diet. I was 10 years old and joined my mum at a local slimming group – in those days it hadn't dawned on anyone that a slimming group might not be the best place to teach a 10-year-old about healthy eating! Having come from a family of yo-yo dieters who loved their food and lived to eat, it seemed a perfectly natural place for me to be – I thought I was destined to be another 'fatty' in the family and so my own yo-yo dieting career began.

I have to say I wasn't very good at it. I suppose I thought just turning up each week would be enough. Why wouldn't it be? After all, I wasn't fat because I ate too much and didn't take part in sport – it was my fate! So again, it felt natural for me to be shamed at my weekly meetings by having to wear a 'piggy mask' for the duration of the class because I'd put on more weight. I was not only destined to be fat, but also to believe I was completely unable to do anything about it! I was caught in my own 'diet trap'.

I think it took another 15 years of repeating the cycle

of being on and off a diet, fluctuating between fat and thin, before I realised that maybe it wasn't fate, and maybe I could do something to break out of the diet prison. My journey towards Diet Freedom had begun ...

It was a very quick and, when I think back, unbelievably easy decision. Within three months I had given up my career in the catering industry, and was enrolled on a course of five years' study to qualify as a state -registered dietitian. The more I learned about food, health and weight the more I was puzzled that, if all this science made sense to someone like me, why was it so hard for people to put into practice?

Why were killers like obesity, heart disease, cancer and diabetes on the increase when simply changing what we eat could prevent them?

That was when another piece of the diet jigsaw slotted into place – people are caught in their own diet trap for reasons that are far more complex than greed, sloth, complacency or ignorance. A whole host of other influences control the choices we make, keeping us caught in the yo-yoing cycle and usually making us feel miserable.

Simply telling us what's good for us isn't enough. If we are going to break free from our diet trap, then changes to the way we eat have to be **sustainable and permanent**. They have to be **realistic and achievable** and, most importantly, they have to be **our own choices**.

After working as a clinical dietitian within the NHS and in research and industry, I decided to set up my own nutrition consultancy to pursue the type of dietetics that interested me the most – preventative, permanent, realistic nutrition that empowers people to get what they want from life!

When I first met Tina and Deborah, my co-authors on this book, I think we all breathed a huge sigh of relief. Fate had brought together three people with a combined total of 90 years of 'diet trap' history, who also had the right combination of knowledge, research, skills – and a passionate enthusiasm to make a difference. We were a combination of ex-serial dieters, natural cooks, avid diet and nutrition researchers, and a chef turned registered dietitian specialising in weight loss, eating disorders and hormone imbalances. The result? We set up an organisation called Diet Freedom and developed a low glycaemic load diet which forms the basis of this book.

Diet Freedom's GL Diet is a simple programme that uses a food selection system based on science: on fact, not fad. It is healthy, not harmful; varied, not restrictive. But, most of all, it's been designed to be *practical and easy* to follow.

We created the programme after lots of painstaking research. We all had different interests in the 'low carbohydrate' phenomenon. I was cautious and very opposed to such a restrictive and unhealthy approach to weight loss. Deborah and Tina had tried the low-carb diet themselves, studied all the plans and talked to many low carbers to understand both the benefits and problems they experienced. This led them to move on, first to the low Glycaemic Index (GI) diet. Then, owing to the GI's complexity and inability to give 'the full picture', they focused their attentions on the low Glycaemic Load (GL) approach – simplified for everyday use. (Please see Chapter One for a full explanation of GI and GL.)

This diet plan has been years in the making for all of us, and the results of our findings are gathered in this book. *The GL Diet* has involved masses of research, recipe development, diet trials on friends, relatives and lots of 'diet trap' victims (you can read about their weight-loss successes throughout this book), weekly meeting trials within health clubs, plus a lot of blood, sweat and tears! We hope you like it as much as we do. It incorporates everything we believe in: delicious, healthy food and flexible eating that has a sound scientific base and a simple format that is easy for everyone to use. By following the GL Diet you will lose weight, keep it off and be healthy. You really don't have to be a 'prisoner' of your diet any more – you WILL escape your diet trap and find your own Diet Freedom.

Nigel Denby
Registered Dietitian
RD BSc Hons

'I attended an eight-week course of Diet Freedom classes and lost half a stone. Best of all, I have found it easy to maintain the loss, as I now know what to eat. I had never managed to lose the weight I gained after my second child – and, to be honest, I was very sceptical at first. I have a busy lifestyle as a teacher and working mum, but I found the diet easy to follow and packed lunches are no problem. As a vegetarian I was really pleased to find loads of vegetarian recipes, which are very good – I have used them a lot. My thighs were the first part to slim down. I lost 10cm very quickly and there is no wobbling now! The most amazing thing for me was that, after only a short time on the diet, I no longer craved crisps, chocolate or puddings. I now have a lot more self-confidence and feel so much better! I dragged a few of my teacher friends to the classes and they too have lost weight.'

*Becky S, Manby, Lincs*

# Why Low GL?

Science – and therefore food science – is constantly evolving. So, to understand the origins of the diet plans that exist today, here's a quick recap of recent popular diet history.

## LOW CALORIE

Until the carbohydrate revolution the low-calorie diet was THE standard, acceptable way to lose weight. The theory was that, if we eat more calories than we burn off, we will put on weight. Well, yes and no. Calories are just one of the contributing factors in weight gain – but certainly not the whole picture. While we can't realistically expect to consume 5,000 calories a day, not exercise and then lose weight, what a calorie-controlled diet doesn't take into account is the fat-storing ability of specific carbohydrates due to their direct effect on our blood glucose and insulin levels.

Balancing blood-glucose levels and preventing the highs and lows caused by eating poor-quality, fast-acting carbohydrates has now been scientifically proven to be a crucial dietary factor, not only in relation to weight gain but also for keeping us healthy full stop. The result of the sharp rise and sudden fall in your blood-sugar levels after eating fast-acting carbs such as a baked potato or a doughnut quickly leads you to crave more of the same fast-acting, glucose-producing foods to make up for the fall. This can leave you ravenously hungry and desperately craving another glucose-producing food fix.

When we eat high-glycaemic foods (ones that quickly deliver glucose to the bloodstream), we have a rapid increase in glucose, or a 'spike'. This prompts our bodies to produce insulin (the most powerful hormone in our bodies, so it isn't to be underestimated). Insulin comes rushing in to flush the glucose out of our bloodstream (if it didn't, we would become very ill, very quickly) and into our liver and muscles, where it is stored for later use as energy. However – and this next bit is crucial – if we constantly eat foods that produce glucose, then we have a continual 'over-supply' of it once the liver and muscles can't store any more. Bearing in mind that the glucose has to be removed from the bloodstream for our safety, it is sent for storage in our fat cells – which is why they, and we, expand if we continue to eat high-glycaemic foods. Obviously, if we expended huge amounts of energy, we would use up a lot of this stored glucose, but sadly the marathon runners among us are in a minority. So, balancing blood-sugar levels and not eating foods that cause the highs and lows is the best way to lose weight.

Dieters rigidly counting their calories might assume that they should be eating foods like rice cakes (low calorie, no fat) in order to lose weight. But they would be wrong. Why? A rice cake is highly processed, for a start, and rice has a higher glycaemic response (a faster rise in your blood-glucose level soon after eating it) than most other foods. These two elements combined mean that a rice cake provokes a moderate to high blood-sugar rise after eating it – so it can actually promote fat storage, despite being low calorie and low fat!

As soon as you eat foods with a high GL, your body turns from a fat-burning engine to a fat-storing machine!

## LOW FAT

We have all been brainwashed into thinking that fat is the monster that will kill us all. In fact, some fats are actually very good for us. Consensus of opinion now based on years of research is that it's fine to eat a diet moderate in fat, providing it's based mainly on the good fats such as olive oil. A diet rich in olive oil is undisputedly a good diet for your health – think Mediterranean diet – so extremely low fat or no fat is generally not a good idea for weight loss or any other aspect of your health. In fact, the 'very low-fat' diet is now obsolete, as it fails to take into account the important distinction between high and low 'Glycaemic Load' carbohydrates (more of that later). And besides, a very low-fat diet is unpalatable to most people.

One extremely negative side effect of the 'very low-fat' diet phenomenon was that we all started to consume huge quantities of low-fat products that were high in sugar, owing to the fact that many manufacturers replaced the fat with sugar to improve the taste and texture.

Science has shown that eating huge quantities of sugar

is not good for us and can cause the unhealthy, unbalanced blood-sugar levels we are trying to avoid. Recent, widely reported studies on rats that consumed large amounts of sugar found that, once the sugar was removed from their diets, they displayed various withdrawal symptoms similar to those displayed by a human experiencing 'cold turkey'. Sugar has also been shown to markedly reduce the effectiveness of our bodies' immune responses – another good reason to minimise our intake!

Trying to lose weight the low-fat way also caused several other problems. One of the worst was the massive increase in the use of highly processed hydrogenated fats, or trans fats, in products – now strongly linked to heart disease and cancer. 'Throw out the butter and buy this healthy, low-fat spread (full of hydrogenated fats)' was the message – when the truth is that a small amount of butter, despite being saturated fat, would actually be better for you.

Many low-fat spreads, chocolate bars, biscuits and processed foods still contain hydrogenated fats/trans fats, although owing to the recent negative research findings manufacturers are now being strongly pressurised to remove them from their products. A good reason to check food labels before you buy.


## LOW CARBOHYDRATE

The 'carbohydrate revolution' became mainstream via Dr Atkins, a pioneer and someone not afraid of standing up to the establishment, which can only be to his credit.

This was indeed a good thing, as he introduced the

importance of 'carbohydrate management' – a critical message we are now finding out as the scientific wheels continue to turn. But Dr Atkins's message focused purely on the **total amount** of carbohydrates we consumed each day, irrespective of which foods they came from. (The importance of this is explained in the Low GI section below.)

Undoubtedly the low-carb diet works – you will lose weight. But, as soon as you make a slip and increase your carbs, you can pile weight back on at an alarming rate. It can also be extremely restrictive and, for many people, an unpalatable regime that cannot be sustained. The first few weeks of pleasure feasting on steak, bacon and eggs, butter and cheese quickly subsides and the craving for fruit and protein-delivery foods such as bread soon takes over and can prove overwhelming.

As yet we don't know the long-term effects of eating a diet based largely on protein and very high in saturated fats. So, until we do, it's best to stick with the olive oil and a small amount of saturated fat – plus a good variety of proteins and different-coloured fruit and vegetables.

## LOW GI

So what is wrong with just taking the total carbohydrates into account and lumping them all together? The Glycaemic Index (GI) of carbohydrate-containing foods has been scientifically tested on human volunteers around the world, and thanks to this research we now know that not all carbohydrates are equal. In fact, they all have very different effects on our all-important blood-glucose and insulin levels. Both low-carb and low-glycaemic diets are similar in that they are based on the effects of carbohydrates on our glucose and insulin levels. But the advantage of following a low-glycaemic diet is that it is based on scientific tests of each *individual* carbohydrate, rather than treating them all the same, as per low-carb plans.

If we want to be slim and healthy, we need to base our diet on foods that have been tested as having a low-glycaemic response, as listed further on in this book. We need to eat the **good carbohydrates** that will supply us with a steady, constant amount of energy and not produce an overload that will be stored as fat.

Balance is key. A healthy diet based on a delicious, varied low-glycaemic food selection plan with moderate exercise is the best we can do for our physical health. It also benefits our mental health – unbalanced blood-sugar levels are linked to Premenstrual Syndrome (PMS), Polycystic Ovary Syndrome (PCOS), depression and mood swings.

## LOW GL

The Glycaemic **Load** (GL) is the final part of the jigsaw, and the focus of this book. Testing for the Glycaemic Index (GI) of foods is a fantastic breakthrough, but it only gives half the true picture. It compares 50g of useable carbohydrates within each food to give us the food's numerical index and decide if it has a high, moderate or low Glycaemic Index.

But what the GI rating of a food doesn't take into account is the average portion sizes we actually eat at meal times OR how many carbs there are in an average portion.

The Glycaemic Load (GL) is derived from a mathematical equation developed by Professor Walter Willett, the highly respected Chairman of the Department of Nutrition at Harvard Medical School. It is based on the GI but also factors in the carb content of an average portion – or the amount of each food we would normally eat at one sitting.

In other words, the GL breaks the science down into a more user-friendly, more accurate reference we can use in everyday life.

We explain exactly how the GL is worked out in the Glycaemic Load – The Facts section (pages 8–12), but for your convenience we have listed all the low-GL foods in Chapter 4.

## FORGET THE FADS!

Finding out the glycaemic response of foods after consumption has been described as the most important change in nutritional thinking in the last 50 years. Forget fads, use the scientific facts. We have moved on from the quantity of carbs to the *quality* of them, and the good news is that you will find a lot of foods that have a high-GI rating are actually low GL – such as carrots, watermelon, sweetcorn and many more. So using the more accurate GL as a reference also equals more food choices! Now, at last, you can confidently make healthy food selections from all food groups and have a nutritious, sustainable, varied and enjoyable way of eating – for ever! AND lose weight as a welcome side effect!

## GLYCAEMIC LOAD – THE FACTS

If you are well versed in the popular weight-loss plans of the last few years – the low-glycaemic approach is now acknowledged as a healthier, more balanced and less restrictive diet than the typical high-protein, high-fat, low-carb regime that has created so much media interest in the effects of carbohydrates. Two years ago the GI was virtually unheard of in the UK, although steadily growing in popularity in Australia, where Professor Jennie Brand Miller, of the University of Sydney, is a pioneer of glycaemic research.

The concept has been around for over 20 years but, partly due to recent positive research and recommendations from Harvard University, it has now reached the mainstream. As such, dietitians, diabetes organisations and doctors are now sitting up and taking notice of this important scientific reference to gauge our body's response to the carbohydrates we consume. It not only has positive implications for obesity, but also for heart health, diabetes and cancer prevention.

So how do scientists test for the GI of each food and what do the results mean? **If the science bit bores you rigid, then move on to Chapter 2 to get started!**

After an overnight fast, scientists feed 10 healthy volunteers with a quantity of food (pasta) that contains 50g of useable carbohydrates. Because the 'carb content' of each food varies considerably, so does the amount of food that testers have to consume to reach the 50g mark. With high-carb foods, such as pasta, they would have to eat a fairly small amount to consume 50g of carbs; but with low-carb foods, such as an apple, they would need to consume a large quantity. Blood samples are then taken at 15- to -30 minute intervals over the next two hours to ascertain the volunteers' blood-sugar and insulin responses to the tested food. This is compared with their response when given 50g of pure carbohydrate (glucose). Each food is then given a numerical index. The Glycaemic Index (GI) ranges from less than 55 (low) to over 70 (high). But don't worry, you don't need to remember this.

You may have seen some GI ratings in popular diet books, but, as we have learned, the GI reference in itself doesn't actually translate to what we eat every day. Why? Well, very simply, it doesn't take into account the portion sizes that we normally eat.

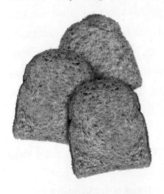
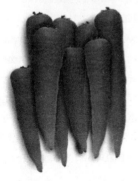

For instance, the amount of bread containing 50g of carbs is about three slices, so that is the quantity volunteers would consume. But to get 50g of carbs from carrots, they would need to eat almost 1½ lbs (0.7kg) of carrots! Unless you are a donkey, you probably wouldn't be consuming that amount at one sitting! Maybe 100g would be nearer the mark.

So, how do we find out what the glycaemic response of a normal-sized 100g 'portion' of carrots would be? Well, that's the easy bit. We have worked it all out for you, so all you need to do is choose from the low-GL food lists provided in Chapter 4. But for those who want to work it out for themselves, here's how to calculate the GL of a food:

Take the GI rating (for example, carrots have an average glycaemic index of approximately 75, which is classed as being high) then divide that number by 100 (75 divided by 100 = 0.75). Then multiply that number by the actual carbohydrates in the portion. So, a 100g portion of carrots would contain approximately 7g of carbs. 0.75 x 7 = a GL of 5.25.

A normal 'portion' of carrots at 5.25 actually has a *very low* GL, so ENJOY – they are good for you and won't make you store fat. If, on the other hand, you had just looked at the GI rating for carrots, 75, you would have assumed they have a high glycaemic index and should be avoided. You may even have read 'DON'T eat carrots – they have a high GI and will make you put on weight.' On the contrary, they are extremely nutritious and they have a low glycaemic **load** per portion – and it's the **load** that counts!

Watermelon is another example of a food that has a high GI but a low GL. It scores highly on the GI, at 72, but bear in mind that testers would have to consume enough of it to reach the 50g carb-content reference level. This equates to eating a whole watermelon, which isn't something we would normally do at one sitting. We are more likely to have a 'portion' of watermelon, and a normal portion size of 120g contains only 6g of carbs. So the GL of watermelon works out at only 4.32 per portion, which means it is a very low-GL food to be enjoyed!

The same goes for many other foods that have a high GI overall but a low GL per average-sized 'portion' – which means more delicious food choices. So, if you have been following a low-GI diet, you will find our low-GL plan far less restrictive and more accurate!

---

**The GL range** is:
**Low GL** 10 or less
**Med GL** 11–19
**High GL** 20 plus

---

**Don't worry about remembering this** – you don't need to. The food lists and guidance in this book will tell you what foods are low GL, based on an average-sized portion. We trust you to estimate what an average-sized portion is. We wanted to avoid weighing and measuring as it is boring and time consuming and, providing you don't confuse 'average' with 'super-sized', it isn't really necessary with the low-GL method.

The Glycaemic Index can also be misleading in that some foods have a low index but a high load.

Most pasta, for instance, has a GI of less than 55, so it is classed as a low-GI food. But the GL of a 180g portion of pasta is between 14 and 24, and so each 'portion' has a moderate to high GL. This is why we advise you to eat it only occasionally and to have a smaller amount (approximately 100g) as an accompaniment rather than use it as the basis of a meal. Have butter beans, couscous or chickpeas instead – they all have a low GL.

We now know that the GL gives a fuller picture and is a more accurate reference than the GI alone – so let's use it in a simplified way to make healthy food selections and lose those stubborn wobbly bits we'd all really rather not have!

**The GL range** or total **Glycaemic Load** per day is:
**Low GL** – less than 80 (which is roughly the amount you will be consuming by using the food lists and following the guidelines)
**High GL** – more than 120 (which is probably what you are consuming now, if you have some weight to get rid of!)

**Just remember:**
**filling carbs not fattening carbs!**

'I've lost 7½ stone (48kg) stone using the Diet Freedom GL Diet plan. It is the most logical approach to losing weight I have found. This way of eating becomes second nature. It makes you feel really good, and so maintaining that weight loss isn't difficult. It has had a really positive impact on the family as well – they have lost weight as a knock-on effect, and we all feel so much healthier and more energetic. With a child in nursery you expect to get a few bugs coming home on a fairly regular basis, but we have also noticed that minor ailments such as colds seem to be a thing of the past.'

*Joanne P, West Sussex*

# 2

# Let's Get Started!

All the tips in this section will sound just like common sense to you. But the chances are that, if your past weight-loss efforts have resulted in you falling off the wagon and quickly returning to bad habits, you may not have 'prepared' well enough to avoid the pitfalls. It isn't *willpower* that is the key to weight loss but *preparation and organisation*. Remember – if you repeat your old ways, you'll get the same old results.

How often have we all started a diet or a mission to get fit, only to find that after a day or two our efforts have fallen by the wayside and we're back to square one? And that left us feeling miserable; like a failure and generally hopeless.

For us, it took years of being trapped in the cycle of recovering from yet another failed diet and preparing to launch on to the next crazy regime for us to realise, 'Wait a minute! Maybe it's not me that's the failure – maybe it's the diet!' This breakthrough moment was like switching on a light, and for the first time we became aware of the fact that we actually never wanted to diet and that we hated diets!

What we *did* want was a way of eating and living which was:

- easy
- delicious
- good fun
- didn't leave us feeling like we were living in purgatory!

That's why we decided to develop the GL Diet, and now we're sharing our experiences and knowledge with you.

It still means that, to break out of the diet trap and find diet freedom, a few changes will have to happen. But before you try and change something, it's usually good to know exactly what needs to change. We found it very helpful to spend a couple of days recording what we eat and drink. This helped us to see which areas of our diets needed work, and we suggest you try it too. You may well start to see patterns: maybe you graze all day on refined carbohydrates, chasing your roller-coaster blood sugars; or maybe you go for long periods without eating at all, making up for it later with huge portions or loads of sugary snacks.

Here are some really practical tips to help you get focused on what needs to change and how to make those changes turn into a permanent part of your life.

## SET SMART GOALS

Often we fail when we diet because we lose touch with what is realistic, or never even get round to starting to change. Once you have decided which areas of your diet you want to work on, set your self SMART goals – they will help to make sure your changes become reality and stay that way.

| SMART GOALS ARE: | | | |
|---|---|---|---|
| Specific | 'I'm going to eat breakfast' | NOT | 'I should eat regularly' |
| | 'I'm going to plan a fruit snack mid-morning' | NOT | 'I'll cut down on biscuits at my tea break' |
| Measurable | 'I'm going to walk for 20 minutes at lunch time, and use the loo on the next floor at work' | NOT | 'I need to exercise more' |
| Achievable | 'I'm going to reduce my alcohol intake to two glasses of wine on weekend nights only' | NOT | 'I'm giving up wine' |
| Realistic | 'When I go out to eat, I'll remember to follow the tips in the Eating Out chapter' | NOT | 'I can't go out for dinner, I'm on a diet!' |
| Time specific | 'I'm going to start changing my life with the GL Diet today!' | NOT | 'That sounds really interesting, I might give it a go one day' |

Work out what will help you be successful and what might get in your way. Use a scale of 1–10 to rate your confidence level: if 0 = no confidence and 10 = total confidence, decide how confident you feel right now. Do you feel you can achieve all your goals with the GL Diet? If not, what will help increase your confidence and make your confidence rating 10? Maybe you could start the plan with a friend or your partner. Maybe you don't shop very regularly and you need to get more organised. Maybe you're worried about the food the rest of the family eats. Maybe you're worried that, if you don't see instant results, you'll give up.

As soon as you work out what you need to be successful, the solutions start to fall into place. The following suggestions might help:

- Find a friend who you know won't try to sabotage your plan, someone who understands that changing can be tough to start with, and agree to support each other.

- Everyone can eat low GL – it's not a diet, it's a long-term, healthy lifestyle change.

- Set yourself some milestones that you can achieve sooner rather than later – such as losing your first half-stone (3kg) and getting into those jeans that right now you can only wear on 'slim days'!

- Get organised. If you were moving house, or starting a new project at work, would you just wake up that morning and think, 'OK, well let's have a go at this'? Of course not!

- If you are going to make successful, permanent changes to the way you eat and live, you have to do some planning. It doesn't have to turn into a military operation, but at least decide what you are going to need to eat for a few days. Select the sort of foods you want for breakfast, lunch and snacks from the meal guides in Chapter 5. Then choose a few recipes from Chapter 6. Or plan your own main meals using the low-GL food lists in Chapter 4. Make a shopping list, buy the food, then eat it – simple!

## Be prepared to make mistakes

This diet plan is not about being perfect all of the time. Sometimes you might choose to eat something you know isn't going to help you reach your goals – we are all human! Other times you might genuinely make a mistake. After all, it took years to develop your current eating habits, and it will take practice to change them – so the odd slip here and there on the route to a new way of eating is only to be expected.

Times like this are called lapses. A *relapse*, however, is a return to your old ways, and the art is to prevent the lapse from turning into a relapse! Lapsing is a normal part of changing, and something we all do. The important thing is to understand why you lapsed – perhaps you forgot to have breakfast and got too hungry, or you didn't take your fruit snack to work and gave in to sugary biscuits. It's not about willpower, it's about learning a new way of eating, and all you did was forget – give yourself a break and learn from it!

Don't let your past dieting experience put you off starting the GL plan. That's the whole point: this isn't a diet and so it won't be the same as any bad dieting experience you may have had in the past. The food isn't boring, no one is going to humiliate you for slipping up, and the eating plan is based on sound scientific evidence. No fads, no crazy ideas, just great food, good advice and superb results.

So now we understand that sometimes a lapse is just the

> Remember: If you do what you always did, you'll get
> what you always got.

result of forgetting that we are choosing to eat healthy
food and feel and look great. But what about when the
effort feels like it's just too much? We all have our food
weaknesses – chocolate? Crisps? Pastry? Desserts? Well,
we've got some fantastic GL Diet-friendly recipes and
suggestions to help you still enjoy a lot of these foods.
But sometimes the environment we're in puts less GL-
friendly food right under our nose and if it's before lunch
or at the end of hard day this can be really tricky. The
answer? You've guessed it BE PREPARED!

## TEMPTATION TAGS …
## FOR WHEN TEMPTATION STRIKES!

We're going to talk about the power of positive thinking
in a moment. Here are some things you can say to yourself,
either in your head or out loud if it helps, for when you
look at tempting food – in the fridge, in the supermarket,
at the petrol station, on a menu, or anywhere temptation
lurks. You can just choose any 'temptation tag' you like –
one that you can remember and one that strikes a chord.
Or you could write a few down and keep them in your
purse, wallet or handbag. Before reaching for the biscuits,
chocolate bar or Cornish pasty, pause for a second, say
your memorised tag – or read your temptation tag from
your list – and then decide whether or not you should buy
it. This really helps you to stop acting on impulse and to
think of the consequences before you grab.

Here are a few ideas. See which works for you and strikes a chord. If you have any other tag ideas, or ones that you find work well, let us know by contacting us at our website (www.dietfreedom.co.uk). It may help someone else!

'I only eat healthy food – not junk food.'
'Will it make me feel better? – no, worse.'
'Junk food equals bigger clothes.'
'Big portions equals bigger clothes.'
'Bad for me – bad for my belly/bum!'
'No thanks – I'm feeling great today'
'Kitchen pickers wear bigger knickers!'
'I'm really not interested in feeling bad any more.'
'No gluttony equals no guilt.'
'Just one will be the tip of the iceberg.'

## GET ACTIVE!

The evidence is overwhelming: a balanced diet combined with moderate exercise is the best thing we can do for our bodies. Here are some pretty convincing reasons why:

- Exercise boosts the immune system, banishing those sniffles and bugs.
- Exercise releases endorphins – the 'feel good' chemicals – into the blood, so it's a natural 'high'.
- Exercise boosts brainpower and memory, so no more embarrassing 'Er…?' moments!
- Exercise is well known to help you sleep better.
- Exercise helps lower the risk of cancer, heart disease, high blood pressure, and so on.

- Exercise can really help you beat cravings and addictions to nicotine, sugar and other drugs.
- Exercise helps you to build an all-important positive self-image – a physical, mental, emotional and spiritual foundation for your growing self-esteem.

So, plan some time to get active. You don't have to go to the gym or start aerobic classes, but do look at your day-to-day routine and see where you could introduce more action. For instance, are there times you could walk instead of driving? Perhaps you could get off the bus a few stops earlier, use the stairs more often, or get the garden sorted? Let's look at it another way – what do you do anyway that counts as exercise?

- Washing the car
- Dusting (with stretches)
- Vacuuming (with vigour)
- Mowing the lawn
- Weeding
- Digging
- Using stairs (instead of lifts or escalators)
- Chasing the kids!

Anything that gets you moving about and feeling a bit warmer will make a difference. Aim for about 20–30 minutes of more energetic activity than you do at the moment, starting off gently then building up slowly.

What do you enjoy?

- Swimming
- Yoga
- Golf
- Dancing
- Weight training
- Sex
- Cycling
- Aerobics
- Walking the dog (if you don't have one, rescue centres are always looking for volunteers – and you'll make a dog's day!)

What have you always wanted to try?

- Belly dancing
- Tai chi
- Aqua aerobics
- Salsa
- Kick-boxing
- Gymnastics
- Tap dancing
- Skipping
- Trampolining

Becoming more active will help boost your weight loss and health. But remember – always take advice from professionals before embarking on any exercise routine, and talk to your doctor first if you have any concerns.

## PLAN HOW YOU WILL CELEBRATE YOUR SUCCESS

Think about all the things you would like to achieve, for example:

- Lose weight
- Have more energy
- Feel happier about your shape
- Feel good on the beach

Decide how you are going to measure your success and how you would like to celebrate each time you hit a milestone on the way to your goals. You might choose big or small celebrations – some new clothes, a day at a health spa, a long hot bath, or a night out. Start positively – book appointments with yourself to celebrate.

## WATCH OUT FOR OLD TRIGGERS!

Chances are that you already have an idea of your danger times – times when it gets all too tempting to raid the chocolate cupboard, or hit the biscuit barrel. Take some time now, when you feel calm, confident and certain you will be successful. Start to think of some strategies, to help you steer clear of your old triggers.

You might decide to clear the cupboards of the foods you want to avoid – although this isn't always possible for people with a family around. Sometimes removing yourself from the trigger situation for a few minutes can help – go for a walk, have a bath or a shower, or phone a friend. Whatever works for you is the right answer, but you are far more likely to find the answer by planning for the rough times during the good times.

If you are still procrastinating – finding every possible reason why you can't manage to change the way you eat to get what you want and be healthy – ask yourself a question: Do you really want your goals enough? If the answer is yes, then make it a big, positive YES and get started with us today.

## KEEPING GOING WITH POSITIVE THINKING

As the weeks go by, we are all highly likely to come up against challenges and moments of self-doubt, no matter how well we are doing. So this is as good a time as any to discuss positive thinking – and its darker sister, self-sabotage.

So far you have all shown amazing strength in overcoming the temptations that day-to-day living throws in your path, even if you think you haven't! There are tools we can use to steer us towards our goals, and a healthy body, without compromising our enjoyment of food.

First, a few words about that very unpredictable thing – our brain. It has many guises and voices, and a good trick is to learn which are helpful, then use those to replace the ones that are unhelpful. People with weight issues tend to think about their physical weight constantly – it's easy to become obsessed with losing weight and focus on it all the time. These thoughts are often accompanied by constant 'internal chatter'.

We all have inner voices. Unfortunately, a lot of the time these 'voices' are critical and unsupportive. Internal critics, martyrs, perfectionists, pleasers, worriers ... We all have them in our heads! Does this 'voice' sound familiar, for instance?

*'When have you ever been successful at losing weight
and keeping it off?'*
*'You're a failure'*
*'Anyone who knows you will just think – oh no, not
another diet. I wonder how long this one will last?'*
*'Start tomorrow – it's not going to work anyway, so you
may as well put it off.'*

Definitely not a good voice! It's critical and destructive –
altogether negative.

A really great start is to encourage yourself and ignore
any negative chatter. Replace the negative words that
come into your mind with positive phrases that you can
use daily. So next time those voices come to pester you,
you can silence them with confidence:

*'I don't have the time.'*
'My health and happiness are important – I'll make
time.'
*'My family won't like the food I have to eat on this diet.'*
'Oh yes they will as it's not "diet" food!'
*'I have to look after everyone all the time, and please
everyone, or they won't like me any more.'*
'People who have the confidence to do things for
themselves are magnetic!'

Do you criticise your own attempts at doing something
and think someone else could have done the job better?
Do you worry about what everyone thinks about you all
the time?

You cannot please everyone. Start to think more about what you need and want from your life. Once you take the first small step to being just you, and not what you think everyone expects you to be, you will find life much easier – and food will become a manageable and less all-encompassing part of your life.

The theory is, we are all born with a unique personality and a mind that is set up to protect that personality and physical body in whatever way it can. As children we learn and develop our defences, which protect us from being vulnerable. For example, we find that our parents and other grown-ups like certain behaviour. So we often bring out that part of ourselves to attain maximum acceptability. And it works, so we keep on doing it while often bottling things up without realising it. As time moves on, we develop different ways of dealing with the aspects of our personality that are suppressed. Some people overeat, drink excessively, turn to drugs, become stressed or become obsessive about certain things. It can become a vicious circle.

Anyone who has experienced the highs and lows of binge eating can recognise how we feel when our eating gets out of control. Once the binge is over, the critical inner voice will remind us of it again and again – which lowers our self-esteem even further and can lead to depression.

With this diet we can and *will* change these negative patterns and lose weight, while increasing our confidence and self-esteem at the same time. This enables us to control our own eating behaviour and to get rid of the emotional and physical weight that has been pulling us down for too long.

There are some very simple steps we can take to change destructive mental dialogue. Be prepared for your 'voices' and reject them! It's amazing how powerful you will feel when you do this.

You can very easily distinguish between your critical inner voice and your own true voice. If you are being hard on yourself, beating yourself up about things, try to remember – it's not you, it's just that scared, judgemental, narrow-minded, protectionist inner voice trying to make you feel bad.

The following method of silencing negative inner voices may sound a little unconventional but it is a widely used coaching tool.

Rather than try to suppress the negative voices, a good trick is to distance them. If you can hear a negative voice yelling into your left ear and seeming very close, it's hard to ignore it. However, if you move that voice further away, so it comes from a distance – the tip of your shoe perhaps – it's not quite so overbearing, is it? Then, if you change the tone of that voice and make it quieter, faster – more of a gabble – and give it a squeaky tone, like it had been sucking helium, or perhaps a quack tone, like Donald Duck ... Suddenly, rather than threatening and overbearing that voice becomes laughable. It's ridiculous, and bears no weight whatsoever. You're free of it! Have a go at this next time your inner voice appears and starts sounding negative – it really works!

To completely silence any leftover nonsense the voices might throw up, tell them how great you feel, how you are becoming more and more confident. They'll soon disappear. They can only stick around if you allow them to – and you do have the power to get rid of them once and for all.

The minute we try and make any change – particularly to our eating pattern – the voices are straight in there to tell us how many times 'diets' have not worked in the past and bombard us with a number of self-sabotage statements. Now that you know how to stifle them with loud, positive statements you can move onwards and upwards.

> Bad habits are broken … Good habits are formed.

As human beings we all have a huge capacity to learn things and store them in our brain's long-term memory. This enables us to recall automatic skills for routine actions: simple procedures such as walking or more complex actions such as driving a car. These skills become automatic because, after lots of repetition and practice, we perform them without conscious thought.

Do you remember how you learned to drive, perhaps, or swim? First by being told how to do it, and then practising yourself until it became second nature. How did that make you feel? Remember how good it felt when you passed your driving test or earned a swimming badge and mastered a skill? Think of any skill you have learned in the past and feel the good feelings of success that went with it.

Now try and remember something you had to unlearn and relearn – driving a different car, a new way of walking after an operation, an alternative route to work after moving house. Would learning a new way of eating or exercising be any different to that?

Our brains have neural pathways, and each habitual action becomes a separate neural pathway, like a short cut. It takes an effort to remember to not take the established route, the short cut, and to lay down a 'new' neural pathway. But, with practice, your brain will establish a new way of doing things, the old pathway will fade, and voila! New habit, new way of eating, new you!

Diet Freedom's GL Diet is about reintroducing the self-respecting, positive, confident voice into your daily life and you wouldn't be reading this book if you didn't have a self-respecting, positive, confident voice – it's that very voice that got you here in the first place! You have taken the biggest step – a great leap forward – because you have taken ACTION. And that in itself is a huge achievement!

Promise yourself three things. I *will*:
- make a habit of doing one thing simply for my own pleasure every day – at least 15 minutes of pure 'me' time;
- put forward an alternative positive scenario to any 'negatives' the silly inner voices come up with … and simply NEVER agree with them;
- start saying 'no' rather than feeling obliged to say 'yes', and make decisions based on what I want and what's good for me.

## THINGS FOR YOU TO THINK ABOUT …

As a child did you have any aspirations that made you stand out from the crowd? What were they? Write them down and think about them. Do you still have a desire to do any of them? If so, try them. You'll be surprised how great you will feel when you do. What things do you *think* you are not particularly good at? How many of those things have you ever actually tried? Try one of them ... Perhaps read about something you are interested in, but have not found time for yet. Investigate that often-thought-about hobby. This is all about you.

Which part of your body did your inner critical voice pick on the most? You know it was blowing it out of all proportion really. It may not have liked your bottom/belly/thighs/upper arms, but you are taking positive action to change this. So realistically, how can it possibly criticise you now.

What do you think you are good at? Admit the things you are secretly proud of! Write them down now, in big bold letters. Picture yourself doing them. How good do they make you feel? Relish that feeling and hold on to it. What do your internal voices squeak about when you decide to lose weight?

When you wake up each morning take a couple of minutes to look in the mirror, smile and say to yourself out loud, in an upbeat and positive tone, 'I am feeling more and more confident each day and, as a result, life is getting better and better!' 'I am enjoying my food AND losing weight. I am finding it easier and easier. I have so much more energy and I feel fabulous!'

Again, it may sound odd but just try it once and then experience how you *feel*. We are not only affected by what others say to us but also by what we say to ourselves. You can really lift your own spirits and *feel* fabulous.

Another good exercise is to lie down and relax. In your mind create a picture of yourself exactly as you would like to be. Imagine every detail – shiny hair, glowing, healthy skin, slim body, radiant with health and feeling very happy. Take a good long, lingering look. Now stop looking and mentally step into the new you. Notice how great that makes you feel inside, how much confidence it gives you, and hold on to that feeling. Try to do this at least once a day – you're preparing your subconscious mind to get used to the new you.

Well done! Congratulations for taking positive action – we will be with you all the way!

---

'I lost a stone (6kg) on the Diet Freedom GL Diet plan. I am very active but, despite exercising, going to the gym twice a week as well as running, I couldn't get rid of the last stone. By changing the foods I was eating I lost a stone over a couple of months and seemed to be eating more food than before. I continue to follow the guidelines and the weight hasn't come back, so I am thrilled, and I've recommended several friends and colleagues to try it. My skin has also improved noticeably and I have had compliments to say I look well and younger!'

*Rena B, Manby, Lincolnshire*

# 3

# How Do I Follow the GL Diet Plan?

We have made it as simple and straightforward as possible. We all have busy lives and we recognise the importance of a user-friendly plan without lots of confusing stages and phases. You won't find any in this book. The GL Diet plan is a permanent life change, so there are no stages, phases or quick fixes! The recipes are basic, quick and don't contain lots of strange ingredients. You don't need to be a Jamie Oliver or a Nigella Lawson to cook them either! For those of us with particularly hectic schedules, there are even speedier ready-made meal suggestions you can buy from the supermarket. So fear not, you can follow the plan even if you have never seen the inside of an oven or, worse still, don't know what one looks like!

Aim for three meals a day and try not to leave more than four hours between eating something – time any snacks to fit in with this four-hour scale if you can. If you go too long without eating, your blood-sugar level will become too low and you may feel the urge to eat anything in sight!

> Breakfast: Choose from the lists in Chapter 5
> Lunch: Choose from the lists in Chapter 5
> Dinner: Choose a recipe from Chapter 6, or a 'fast' meal from the shopping guidelines in Chapter 7

Of course, there will be days when lunch will be your main meal. Feel free to swap and change meals – flexibility is key. Alternatively you can just make up your own meals as you go along, based on the low-GL food lists. Dining out is covered in depth in Chapter 8.

## QUANTITIES

We trust you to have 'average' portions at each meal, and not to 'super-size' them! A good rule of thumb is not to eat more than you could fit into your cupped hands. (At this stage everyone looks at their cupped hands to see how much will fit in – those with bigger hands are smiling!) Think 'satisfied' not 'stuffed'!

## TRIGGER FOODS

Most people have certain 'trigger' foods that make them want to overeat – and generally they are the high-GL ones. You will know what your triggers are (be it chocolate, biscuits, bread, French fries) and they are obviously best cleared from the cupboards and kept out of the house if at all possible.

## MOVE ABOUT MORE

See Chapter 2 for a few ideas on how to get active.

'I have been a diabetic for 11 years, and found managing both my sugars and weight to be time-consuming and sometimes quite difficult. Using the GL, as explained in the Diet Freedom plan GL Diet, has helped a lot. My (blood) sugars are under far better control than they were before, my weight loss has been dramatic, and while the loss is now slowing down it's still coming off as I get closer to my target weight. I am now more motivated to exercise, and am finding that both my energy levels and mood are very positively affected when sticking to the low-GL plan. It is also an easy plan to follow. Dieting has always been a trial, a real pain! But this is simple and gives me the freedom to eat very well and still get healthier. As a great side effect, I need to use less insulin each day than I did before.'

*Gary P (type II diabetic), London*

# 4

# Low-GL Food Lists

## MILK AND CREAM

Providing you are not intolerant of dairy products, small quantities of skimmed or semi-skimmed milk or cream are acceptable. Try and limit it to ¼ pint of milk/unsweetened soya milk and 1 tablespoon of cream or 2 tablespoons of crème fraîche per day. Try not to use low-fat cream alternatives, as they often contain unhealthy hydrogenated/ trans fats and sugar. You can use 'squirty' cream, as it is aerated so you tend to use less, but make sure it is the 100% cream with no added sugar – check the label.

## YOGHURT

Yoghurt is fine, providing it has no added sugar. Greek yoghurt or bio yoghurt are good choices. Go for natural wherever possible.

## CHEESE

Cheese is fine in small amounts. Low-fat cheeses are best and most supermarkets do a good half-fat Edam as well as other varieties. Cottage cheese and natural cream cheeses are also good choices. Full-fat cheeses should be limited, as they are very calorie dense (even on an unrestrictive GL plan you still need to keep an eye on the amount of calorie-dense foods that you eat). As a guide, 75g of half-fat cheese or 50g of full-fat cheese per day are acceptable.

## EGGS

Rightly described as 'nature's perfect food'. Stick to free-range eggs where possible. Recent research from Harvard University suggests one egg per day is acceptable – unless you have been advised otherwise.

## CHOCOLATE

If you want to eat chocolate, have smaller quantities (two or three squares) of high-cocoa chocolate, such as Lindt or Green & Black's Organic, which has 70% or 85% cocoa solids and thus less sugar. It also has a stronger taste so you tend to eat less. We are currently developing healthy chocolate products – bars, shakes and so on – with natural ingredients that have a low GL, so you can eat them without guilt. See www.dietfreedom.co.uk for up-to-date product information. Cocoa is actually very good for you – it's just all the other stuff they add to it that isn't!

## MEAT AND FISH

Buy fresh rather than pre-packaged produce. All meat and fish, in their natural states, are low GL, as they don't contain carbohydrates. Choose natural, unprocessed, lean cuts of meat and fresh fish where possible. Oily fish (tuna, salmon, mackerel, sardines, and so on) are a very healthy choice. Chicken and turkey are great alternatives to red meat, while soya and Quorn can be used as a meat substitute.

## NUTS

Nuts have a low GL and are a healthy food choice in their natural state, so choose natural nuts rather than the salted ones. But they are also very calorie dense, so they should be kept to a minimum – no more than a small handful a day. (If you use ground almonds in cooking, don't forget to include them.) Nuts are a much healthier snack than sugar-filled sweets and biscuits, and are less likely to stimulate food cravings due to their low glycaemic response. The latest research shows that eating a handful of almonds per day actually lowers cholesterol levels. We have found that for a minority of people eating nuts has stalled their weight loss. This may be because it is very easy to eat too many and they tend to come in large bags – so a note of caution there.

## SNACKS

Low-GL fruit or vegetable crudités (see also the dip recipes in Chapter 6) from the food lists make an excellent snack. Small bags of baby carrots are now available from most supermarkets. They are very crisp and sweet, and great to keep in the fridge or at work for those 'I need munchies' moments. Some coffee shops such as Costa now do carrot batons with dips – an ideal snack when out and about. Dried apricots, also available from all supermarkets, are a delicious option for when you want something sweet. Sunflower seeds or mixed-seed snacks are another healthy low-GL snack option. Peanuts are also low GL, so a small bag is fine. Beware the 'natural' bars as they are often full of sugar (even if it's organic brown sugar, it still has the same GL as white sugar).

## SUGAR/SUGAR SUBSTITUTES

Try to avoid sugar as far as possible. We already consume huge amounts of it without realising, as so many processed foods contain various forms of it under different names such as glucose, sucrose and dextrose. Sugar is a cheap ingredient, which is why it is so widely used. High-fructose corn syrup (not to be confused with fructose or fruit sugar) is another form of high-glycaemic sweetener to avoid. Natural and brown sugars have a similar moderate GL to white sugar. Often low-fat products have had the fat replaced with sugar to improve the taste, and even savoury foods are often 'sweetened'. So check your labels and, if sugar or one of its compounds is listed within the first four ingredients, choose something else – it will help to avoid the cumulative effects.

If you need to sweeten food and drinks, fructose (fruit sugar) can be used sparingly as a sugar substitute. Available from most supermarkets, fructose has a lower glycaemic response than sugar and will not raise your blood-sugar levels as quickly. It looks and tastes like sugar but is sweeter so you can use less – make sure you follow the usage instructions on the box. It is also heat stable so it can be used for baking.

Honey has a moderate GL so the odd teaspoon won't hurt. Most artificial sweeteners have a low GL and are found in many products, including low-calorie and sugar-free products. Beware of the polyols (sugar alcohols) such as maltitol, used in some diabetic and diet products – they can have a very potent and immediate laxative effect! The GL of polyols varies and, although it is suggested that the carbohydrates in them 'don't count', as they are metabolised in a different way, the jury is still out on this one.

## BREAD/PASTA/RICE

Choose a low-GL bread such as Burgen, a tasty sliced brown bread containing soya and linseeds, which is now available from most supermarkets. Pumpernickel bread, again widely available, is also a good low-GL choice. While trying to lose weight, only consume small amounts of bread (a maximum of one slice a day for women and two for men). Some people find bread can cause bloating, so, if you feel uncomfortable after eating, it may be better to get your fibre from other sources such as fibrous vegetables, fruit and pulses.

Pasta, while having a fairly low GI, has a moderate to high GL. Higher than bread or potatoes in fact! We recommend that during weight-loss mode you only have it occasionally. If you do indulge, don't overcook it as it raises the GL. Just boil it lightly with added olive oil for a few minutes until cooked al dente. Serve pasta as a side dish instead of making it the main part of the meal. When using pasta in recipes try and keep to no more than 100g (dry weight) per person and use dried or fresh pasta (not tinned). Noodles are usually made from wheat or rice and should be treated in the same way as pasta. Shop-bought pasta sauces vary in the healthiness of their ingredients, so again look for the ones with no added sugar.

Rice has a very high GL, much higher than potatoes, bread and even higher than pasta. Choose extra vegetables and salads instead of rice when possible. You could also substitute it for, or mix it with, pearl barley or couscous – both have a low GL. Bulgar wheat and buckwheat have a moderate GL, so can be used sparingly. If you absolutely have to have rice, choose wild rice, or a long-grain rice such as basmati and keep it to a maximum of two tablespoons (cooked). The GL of rice depends on its amylose content, which is not listed on the label. (Amylose is a type of starch found in the microscopic granules that make up a single rice grain.) A high amylose content equals a lower glycaemic response. The rice with the highest GL is the short-grain rice used in Asian restaurants!

## SALADS

Salads are an excellent and healthy choice, and with so many varieties now available they need never be boring. Make up your own dressings with extra-virgin olive oil, lemon juice, vinegar and fresh herbs and spices – see the dressings recipes on pages 154–55. Research has shown that adding lemon or vinegar will actually reduce the overall GL of a meal – an added incentive to be generous!

## FRUITS

Choose fruit with a low GL from the following list:

Apples

Apricots

Bananas

(the GL increases
substantially when ripe, so
go for the under-ripe green
flecked ones)

Blackberries

Blueberries

Cherries

Figs (fresh only)

Grapes

Grapefruit

Kiwis

(choose firm ones – not
over ripe)

| | |
|---|---|
| Lemons | Peaches |
| Limes | Pears |
| Mandarins | Pineapples |
| Mangoes | Plums |
| Melons | Raspberries |
| Nectarines | Strawberries |
| Oranges | Tangerines |
| Papaya | Ugli Fruit |
| Pawpaw | Watermelon |

Dried fruits such as raisins, sultanas and prunes have a fairly high GL. However, dried apricots/apple/strawberries and raspberries are much lower. Tinned fruits often have added syrup or sugars, so unless they are just in their own natural juices, avoid.

The following unsweetened fruit juices are acceptable if they are 100% fruit, but limit to 120ml maximum per day (add water if you want to make a longer drink):

| | |
|---|---|
| Apple | Grapefruit |
| Orange | Peach |
| Pear | Pineapple |

Juices with 'bits' have a lower GL than plain juices, as they have more fibre and are more like eating the whole fruit.

## VEGETABLES
Choose low-GL vegetables from the following list:

| | |
|---|---|
| Artichoke | Avocado |
| Asparagus | Baked beans (sugar-reduced) |
| Aubergine | Beans (black, butter, garbanzo, |

green, kidney, lima, haricot, pinto, soya)
Bean sprouts
Broccoli
Brussels sprouts
Cabbage
Carrots
Cauliflower
Celery
Celeriac
Chickpeas
Collard greens
Corn on the cob
Courgettes
Endive
Kale
Kohlrabi
Leeks
Lentils
Lettuce
Mangetout
Mushrooms

Okra
Onions
Olives
Parsnips (moderate GL – use sparingly)
Peas (dried, green, yellow or split)
Peppers (red, green, yellow plus hot peppers)
Pickles (sugar-free)
Potatoes (baby new)
Pumpkin
Radishes
Sauerkraut
Spinach
Squash (yellow)
Swede
Sweetcorn
Sweet potatoes (moderate GL – use sparingly)
Tomatoes
Yams (as per sweet potatoes)

If you do buy tinned vegetables, try to find ones with no added sugar.

## GRAINS/BRAN/FIBRE

Buckwheat kasha (moderate GL – use sparingly)
Bulgur wheat (moderate GL – use sparingly)
Couscous
Oat bran

Pearl barley
Rice bran (has a very low GL of 1.5 per 30g)
Porridge oats (steel-cut or old-fashioned oats are best – and they can be microwaved!)

Cereals are generally full of added sugar, so skip them. You can make your own muesli as an alternative (see the muesli recipe on page 53). Or try old-fashioned oat porridge rather than the quick-cook variety.

Fibre is a *crucial* part of a balanced diet and generally the more intact fibre contained in foods the lower the GL. If your diet doesn't include many fibrous foods, we recommend you add psyllium husk to your diet, which is an excellent source of fibre available at health-food shops. Or you could add ground or presoaked linseeds. Both of these must be accompanied by adequate water intake.

## FLOURS

Minimise your use of flour (wheat, corn, potato, and so on) for sauces and baking. Almond flour (ground almonds) is an excellent, healthy substitute to bake with. For thickening savoury and sweet sauces, you can use xanthan gum, a thickener available from most health-food shops. You only need a small amount, whisked into the liquid for best results. Otherwise a teaspoon or so of flour/cornflour won't do any harm.

## CORN PRODUCTS

Corn products (tortilla chips, corn chips, polenta, maize meal, cornstarch, and so on) generally have a high-glycaemic response, so are not a good choice.

## POTATOES AND OTHER ROOT VEGETABLES

The good news is that, in a low-GL diet, some potatoes are OK – unlike most low-GI or low-carb regimes. In fact, they generally have a lower GL than pasta or rice. A few new potatoes are fine. Most smaller, immature or 'baby' vegetables have a lower GL than their fully grown counterparts because of their lower starch content. Sweet potatoes and yams have a medium GL, so use them in small quantities (one medium sweet potato). If you have never tried sweet potatoes, they are delicious – especially when mashed with crème fraîche and black pepper – and also very nutritious. The worst potato choices are French fries, baked potatoes and instant mashed potatoes.

Swede is a good low-GL choice. Parsnips have a moderate GL, so use only sparingly. We talked about carrots earlier in the book – enjoy and eat them often! All types of onions are great, as is garlic. Also see the delicious mash recipe on page 109 – use swede, carrots, celeriac, sweet potatoes or a delicious combination!

'I attended the Diet Freedom course at my health club not to lose weight but to learn about healthy eating. I always thought jacket potatoes were very healthy until I found out the effect they have on your blood sugars. It was the educational aspect that appealed to me. I suffer from Irritable Bowel Syndrome (IBS) but since changing my diet I don't feel at all bloated. I also noticed the mood-balancing effect of changing to lower-glycaemic foods – particularly with improving PMS and stress. Because you can still eat "normal" foods my family are quite happy eating this way and haven't complained at all. There is a lot more to this diet plan than weight loss.'

Jacky B, Grimoldby, Louth, Lincolnshire

# 5

# Low-GL Breakfast and Lunch Lists

The 'you must eat this on day one of week one and this on day two' approach doesn't do it for us – we wanted more choice! Choose what you want from the breakfast and lunch lists. Improvise by swapping things around ... Just make sure that you are choosing a varied diet – lots of different-coloured vegetables and fruits, plenty of fibre and a good variety of protein sources with small amounts of dairy.

## LOW-GL BREAKFASTS

- Bacon and tomato omelette
- Reduced-sugar beans on toasted low-GL bread
- Boiled eggs, with toasted low-GL bread (butter or olive-oil-based spread optional)
- Cheese omelette
- Fruit smoothie made from milk/soya milk and any low-GL fruits
- Grilled bacon with poached egg and grilled tomatoes
- Grilled sausages (high meat content of at least 85% – you can buy 95% meat sausages from most supermarkets and some butchers) on low-GL toasted bread

- Diet Freedom muesli (see Chapter 6 for the recipe – it's delicious!)
- Any melon quarter plus toasted low-GL bread spread with cream cheese
- Low-GL fruits sliced and topped with a tablespoon of plain/sugar-free/bio yoghurt
- Low-GL toasted bread spread with cream cheese and layers of ham and tomato
- Low-GL toasted bread with no-sugar-added peanut butter
- Melted cheese on low-GL toasted bread with sliced tomato
- Mushroom omelette
- Poached eggs with tinned tomatoes on low-GL toasted bread
- Old-fashioned oats (not instant) with water, milk or soya milk plus chopped fresh strawberries (optional)
- Sardines (or any fish) on low-GL toasted bread
- Scrambled eggs with smoked salmon or bacon
- Scrambled eggs on low-GL toasted bread
- Smoked salmon and cream cheese on low-GL toasted bread
- Smoked salmon or tuna omelette
- Sugar-free bran sticks (available from health-food shops) with a small amount of fructose and semi-skimmed/skimmed/soya milk
- Sugar-free jam on low-GL bread
- Swiss cheese, sliced tomatoes and sliced ham
- Two cheese sticks and an apple or pear
- Two halves of grapefruit sprinkled sparingly with fructose and grilled
- Two halves of papaya (pawpaw) with freshly squeezed

lime or lemon juice
- A big slice of watermelon

## LOW-GL LUNCHES

- Any poached fish with salad and dressing
- A medium sweet potato can be quickly cooked in the microwave – serve with your choice of filling and a side salad with olive oil dressing
- Asparagus soup
- Broccoli and stilton soup
- Carrot and coriander soup
- Cauliflower and bacon soup
- Celery soup
- Cheese and tomato salad
- Chicken or turkey salad with olive-oil-based dressing or low-fat mayonnaise
- Chicken soup
- Cottage-cheese salad with olive-oil-based dressing
- Egg salad
- Fish fingers, poached egg and sugar-reduced beans
- Fish soup
- Reduced-sugar baked beans on low-GL toast
- French onion soup (avoid the croutons unless using low-GL bread)
- Ham salad with coleslaw (check any shop-bought coleslaw for sugar content – some are very high)
- Lentil soup
- Mozzarella cheese and beef-tomato slices, layered with balsamic dressing
- Open bacon sandwich with four rashers of grilled bacon on low-GL bread

- Open cottage cheese and tomato sandwich on low-GL bread
- Poached eggs, bacon and tomatoes
- Prawn salad
- Smoked salmon pâté (or smoked mackerel pâté – see the recipe on page 157) on low-GL toasted bread
- Tomato or tomato and basil soup
- Tuna or any oily fish with salad
- Tuna pâté on one slice of low-GL toasted bread

Home-made soups are preferable, or look for natural soups without added sugar, potatoes, pasta or rice. The fresh carton soups tend to have more natural ingredients and less, if any, sugar added.

*A teaspoon of tomato ketchup or brown sauce is fine for the amount of sugar in it.*

In the recipes section, Chapter 6, you'll find some great salads, dips and dressings, which are ideal for lunchboxes. There's also a quiche, a frittata and many other options that are delicious cold. Soups in a thermos will keep winter days warm and are also very filling.

'Because I have a very demanding lifestyle, my main concern is health and energy – although, like anyone, I like to keep an eye on my weight. The Diet Freedom GL Diet has given me the information I need to have the freedom to eat as I choose. As far as overall health is concerned, my energy levels have increased. I also seem to be less bothered by minor ailments and generally need to sleep less.'

*Anders J, E. Sussex*

# 6

# Low-GL Recipes

The vast majority of the recipes in this chapter will take less than half an hour – many of them only 10 minutes! We know you are busy and recognise you want good food that will keep you on track, food that all the family will enjoy and food that is healthy and will help you lose rather than put on the pounds. We have included many delicious vegetarian recipes that can be adapted to include meat. Enjoy! We love to receive feedback, so if you have any comments (good or bad), or your own recipe suggestions, please visit us at www.dietfreedom.co.uk and share your thoughts and inspirations with fellow dieters!

## PASTA

You will see we have included pasta in a few of the recipes, despite it having a moderate to high GL. We have limited the amount to a maximum of 100g per person, so you won't be getting a huge plateful but more of an accompaniment, with healthy vegetables and varied proteins forming the basis of the meal.

## FATS

You can choose lower-fat options of the recipes simply by switching around the ingredients – low-fat cheese instead of full-fat, crème fraîche instead of cream, and so on. Don't forget that olive oil is a 'good' fat, so be generous! Adding vinegar and lemon juice has been shown to actually lower the overall GL of the meal, so get those lovely dressings flowing! We recommend you use olive-oil-based spreads, available from all supermarkets. As a general rule, these contain virtually no trans fats/hydrogenated fats but do always check the labels.

## SWEETENING

We have used limited amounts of fructose in some of the recipes. None of the dessert recipes will be very 'sweet', as the idea is to wean you away from sickly sweet foods. Artificial sweeteners are generally low GL, if you prefer to use them instead, but the results in baking are often poor, leaving a chemical aftertaste. Some of us are seemingly addicted to sugar; the more we eat the more we want. Try to get used to and enjoy the natural sweetness of whole fruits and your body will reward you.

As fibre plays a critical role in the GL of foods, it is far better to eat the peel of fruit instead of removing it. Apple peel, for example, is very fibrous and will slow the absorption of glucose into your bloodstream, lowering its glycaemic effect/GL. Buy organic fruit, where possible and wash skins thoroughly before use.

## SPICES

We love the Seasoned Pioneers range of spice blends.

When you're looking for things to replace salt in your cooking, spices are great fun to experiment with – start with just a pinch so you get used to the flavours first! The Seasoned Pioneers range is available at Sainsbury's and other stores. If you can't find them, visit our website at www.dietfreedom.co.uk and we'll help you track some down.

## ADAPTING RECIPES

Most recipes can be adapted to lower their GL. It just takes a bit of practice and experimenting. Cakes, crumbles and muffins can all be made by substituting white flour with either ground almonds (or other ground nuts such as hazelnuts or walnuts), soya flour, gram flour (chickpea flour), coconut flour (ground desiccated coconut – unsweetened) or whey protein powder (available from health-food shops). You can even make low-GL Yorkshire puds using ground almonds to replace the white flour – they may be a bit stodgier but they taste nice all the same. Use a mixture of these alternative flours or whichever you prefer, although gram flour is better in savoury recipes. Also ground almonds, like most nuts, are extremely high in calories so mixing them with other flour substitutes such as soya flour is a good idea.

In sweet recipes you can use a sugar substitute such as fructose, and as it is sweeter than sugar you can use a lot less of it. Hopefully you will find that, by adding plenty of fruit, such as apples or strawberries, to cakes and muffins, you really don't need much, if any, extra sweetness.

Instead of making mash with white potatoes, use other low-GL vegetables such as carrots, cauliflower, celeriac or swede – whatever your preferred combination (see vegetable side dishes on pages 101–153. They also make great pie toppings. For fish pie, stir in a teaspoon of mustard to give the mash an extra bite. For cottage pie, add a little chilli, or a little grating of horseradish, lots of freshly ground black pepper and a drop of cream – and you have a gorgeous mash that most people will compliment you on without even noticing it isn't made from potato!

Instead of a normal white baked potato, try baking sweet potatoes. They have a moderate GL, though, so don't go too mad! They take less time to bake in the oven or they can be cooked quickly in the microwave. Serve them with delicious toppings such as a little butter or olive-oil-based spread and some grated cheese, or some half-fat cream cheese with a side salad. Sprouted seeds such as chickpeas, sunflower seeds and mung beans are a nice addition – crisp, fresh and very good for you. Or you could serve low-sugar baked beans, home-made chilli con carne, coleslaw – the list is endless.

To make pancakes and batters, once again just substitute the white flour. You can either make sweet pancakes, and squeeze fresh lemon or orange juice over them, or you can fill them with savoury fillings such as cooked chicken pieces, tomatoes, cheese and bacon, ham – whatever you like. You may need to turn the pancakes over carefully with a spatula, as they are slightly more fragile than regular pancakes, but they taste just as delicious.

You can also make your own ice cream using low-GL fruit such as strawberries or raspberries (see dessert recipes on pages 159–174). If you are short of time, choose a quick recipe such as our Quick Strawberry Ice Cream (see page 163).

Chocolate with 70 or 85% cocoa solids can be used whenever a recipe calls for chocolate – you can grate it for decoration or chop it into small pieces and make chocolate chip muffins.

# BREAKFAST

## DIET FREEDOM MUESLI
2 cups old-fashioned porridge oats (don't use the
   microwave quick-cook ones)
¼ cup sunflower seeds
¼ cup linseeds
¼ cup pumpkin seeds
½ cup nut pieces – hazelnuts, almonds, Brazil nuts or
   walnuts (or a mixture)
1 cup sugar-free bran sticks (optional)
skimmed milk or unsweetened soya milk, to serve

If you prefer your muesli 'toasted', follow the instructions below. If not, you can just mix all the ingredients together.

Preheat the oven to 200°C/400°F/Gas Mark 6. Place all the ingredients (except the bran sticks) on a baking tray in the oven for approximately 15 minutes, until the mixture is lightly 'toasted' and the oats have turned golden at the edges. Carefully remove the mix from the oven and allow it to cool. Once cooled, place the toasted ingredients with the bran sticks in a storage jar and shake until mixed well. Adding the optional dried or fresh fruit and coconut below will 'sweeten' the muesli without the need for added sugar, although you could add a teaspoon of fructose if you prefer. Serve with skimmed milk or unsweetened soya milk.

*Optional extras: ¼ cup oat bran, ¼ cup chopped dried apricots, ½ cup dried apples or dried strawberries, ½ cup unsweetened coconut flakes/desiccated coconut. Or you can add chopped fresh low-GL fruit, as desired, just before serving.*

The low-GL breakfast list on page 45–46 provides many breakfast suggestions – we've kept it simple, as this is the way we like it first thing in the morning!

# MAIN MEALS

## Chicken, turkey and duck meals

ASPARAGUS CHICKEN
Preparation time: 15 minutes
Cooking time: 20 minutes
Serves 2

1 teaspoon butter or olive-oil-based spread
2 chicken breasts
8 asparagus spears, cooked and drained
1 tablespoon Dijon mustard
1 medium onion, finely chopped
1 teaspoon tarragon
1 red pepper, deseeded and chopped
125g single cream or crème fraîche
toasted almonds, to garnish

Fry the chicken breasts in the butter or olive-oil-based spread until cooked thoroughly. Add the cream/crème fraîche and bring to the boil. Turn down the heat and stir until the cream has reduced and thickened. In a separate pan, fry the red pepper, asparagus, onions and tarragon until tender. Then transfer this to the pan with the chicken and cream, and add the mustard. Stir until heated through thoroughly. Sprinkle with the toasted almonds and serve.

## CHEESE AND CHIVE CHICKEN

Preparation time: 10 minutes
Cooking time: 20 minutes
Serves 2

2 skinned chicken breasts
50g Double Gloucester cheese, grated
1 heaped teaspoon Dijon mustard
½ bunch chives, snipped into small pieces
low-GL vegetables, to serve

Grill the chicken breasts for about 15 minutes or until well
cooked throughout. Meanwhile, mix together the cheese,
chives and mustard to form a paste. Carefully spread the
paste over the chicken breasts and place under a hot grill
for about 3 minutes or until the cheese has melted. Serve
with low-GL vegetables such as green beans or broccoli.

## CHICKEN KORMA

Preparation time: 10 minutes
Cooking time: 15 minutes
Serves 2

2 chicken breasts, diced*
1 tablespoon extra-virgin olive oil
1 tablespoon mild curry powder
1 tablespoon tomato purée
1 tablespoon ground almonds
½ medium onion, chopped
2 tablespoons single cream or crème fraîche
1 tablespoon water
mixed salad, to serve

Fry the chicken and onions in the olive oil until browned and cooked through. Add the curry powder and fry for 1 minute. Stir in the cream, ground almonds, water and tomato purée, and bring to the boil, stirring continually. Simmer for 2–3 minutes. Serve with a mixed salad.

* Turkey can be used instead of chicken, if preferred

## TURKEY MEATBALLS

Preparation time: 10 minutes
Cooking time: 30 minutes
Serves 2

225g minced turkey
½ tablespoon olive oil
1 onion, finely chopped
1 heaped teaspoon paprika
50g ground almonds
1 egg white
freshly ground black pepper
tomato-based sauce and low-GL vegetables, to serve

Preheat the oven to high. In a pan, heat the oil, add the
onion and cook gently for 10 minutes. Then add the
paprika and fry for 30 seconds. Transfer to a food processor
with the minced turkey, ground almonds and egg white.
Season well and whiz until blended. Form into 8
meatballs, then place them on a baking sheet and cook
them in the oven for 30 minutes. Serve with a tomato-
based pasta-style sauce and low-GL vegetables.

## LIME CHICKEN

Preparation time: 10 minutes
Cooking time: 20 minutes
Serves 2

2 chicken breasts
1 tablespoon extra-virgin olive oil
1 medium onion, finely chopped
1 clove garlic, minced
¼ teaspoon each of chilli powder, ground cumin,
    coriander, turmeric
1 tablespoon soy sauce
juice of 1 lime
low-GL vegetables, to serve

Brown the chicken in the oil over a medium heat. Add the
onion and garlic, and fry for 2 minutes. Then add all the
other ingredients except the lime juice. Reduce the heat,
cover and cook for 20 minutes or until thoroughly cooked
through. Just before serving, pour over the lime juice.
Serve with low-GL vegetables from the food list in
Chapter 4.

## CHICKEN AND FRENCH GREEN BEAN STIR-FRY

Preparation time: 10 minutes
Cooking time: 10 minutes
Serves 2

2 chicken breasts, diced*
1 tablespoon extra-virgin olive oil
½ medium onion, chopped
2 tablespoons tomato purée
2 tablespoons water
2 portions French green beans (or use frozen beans straight
   from the bag)
2 tablespoons single cream/crème fraîche
1 teaspoon chilli powder/paste
freshly ground black pepper
2 teaspoons grated Parmesan cheese, to serve

Stir-fry the chicken and onion in olive oil until browned, making sure the chicken is cooked through. Add the tomato purée, chilli powder, water and black pepper, and bring to the boil, stirring continually. Parboil the green beans and, when they are tender, drain, add to the stir fry and stir in the cream. Sprinkle with Parmesan and serve.

* Turkey can be used instead of chicken, if preferred

## SHAHI CHICKEN
Preparation time: 30 minutes
Cooking time: 30 minutes
Serves 4

500g boneless, skinless chicken breasts, cut into
  2.5cm strips
3 tablespoons extra-virgin olive oil
1 onion, finely chopped
200g tinned chopped tomatoes
50g unsalted cashew nuts
3 garlic cloves, crushed
½ teaspoon garam masala
5cm piece fresh ginger root, finely grated (or 1 teaspoon
  powdered ginger)
¼ teaspoon red chilli powder
¼ teaspoon coriander powder
¼ teaspoon ground turmeric
25ml crème fraîche
broccoli, to serve

Cover the cashews with hot water and soak for 30 minutes. Heat the oil in a saucepan, add the onions and fry until golden brown. Add the garlic, garam masala, ginger, red chilli powder, coriander powder and turmeric to the pan and fry, stirring for 1–2 minutes. Add the chicken and fry for 3 minutes, turning halfway through. Add the tomatoes and mix well. Then reduce the heat, partially cover, and simmer for 20 minutes, turning from time to time until the chicken is tender. Drain most of the water from the cashews, transfer them to a food processor and whiz them to a thick paste. Then add the cashew paste and crème fraîche to the chicken and bring to the boil, adding a little water to give a smooth, slightly thick sauce. Serve with broccoli.

## TURKEY AND SPINACH BAKE

Preparation time: 10 minutes
Cooking time: 30 minutes
Serves 4

500g fresh spinach, washed and chopped
350g cooked turkey, shredded
275g Cheddar cheese, grated
freshly ground black pepper
grated nutmeg (or pinch ground nutmeg)

Preheat the oven to 180°C/350°F/Gas Mark 4 and grease a 25cm ovenproof casserole dish. Place the spinach in the casserole dish and top with the shredded turkey. Season with pepper and nutmeg, and sprinkle with the cheese. Bake for 25 minutes until golden brown.

## CHICKEN FRITTATA

Preparation time: 5 minutes
Cooking time: 45 minutes
Serves 2

2 large chicken breasts
2 tablespoons extra-virgin olive oil
1 red onion, peeled and diced
25g olive-oil-based spread or butter
1 garlic clove, peeled and finely chopped
1 red and 1 yellow pepper, deseeded and finely sliced
6 large free-range eggs
freshly ground black pepper
50g grated Gruyère cheese (or Jarlsberg, Mature
    Cheddar or Parmesan)
peas and side salad, to serve

Preheat the oven to 180°C/350°F/Gas Mark 4. Smear
the chicken breasts with the olive-oil-based spread or
butter, place them on a baking tray and cook them in the
oven for 40 minutes. Allow them to cool, then slice into
strips. Heat the olive oil in a frying pan and sauté the
onion and garlic until softened. Add the peppers and
sauté for 4 minutes. Then add the chicken, the eggs and
seasoning of black pepper. Stir in the Gruyère cheese and
cook over a low heat until just set. Place under the grill
for a few seconds until browned on top. Serve with peas
and a side salad.

## CHINESE CHICKEN

Preparation time: 10 minutes
Cooking time: 10 minutes
Serves 2

1 tablespoon extra-virgin olive oil
2 chicken breasts, finely sliced
4 thinly sliced carrots
1 medium onion, finely sliced
8 button mushrooms, sliced
1 green pepper, thinly sliced
handful bean sprouts
½ teaspoon ground ginger (or 2.5cm piece of fresh
    ginger root, grated)

Heat the oil in a large frying pan. Then add the chicken
and vegetables, and sprinkle with the ginger. Quickly stir-
fry for 5–10 minutes or until the chicken is cooked
through.

# THAI GREEN TURKEY CURRY

Preparation time: 30 minutes

Cooking time: 30 minutes

Serves 4

50g creamed coconut (from a block)

500g diced turkey

1 tablespoon extra-virgin olive oil

175g oyster mushrooms, wiped and sliced

1 red or yellow pepper, deseeded and chopped

2 tablespoons Thai green curry paste

2 tablespoons chopped fresh coriander

coriander sprigs, to garnish

side salad, to serve

Dissolve the creamed coconut in 10 fl oz (0.3 litres) of hot (not boiling) water, stirring until it becomes smooth. Then set it to one side. Next, heat the oil in a large frying pan, or wok, and seal the turkey on all sides. Add the mushrooms and chopped pepper, then continue to sauté for 2 minutes. Add the curry paste and cook for a further 2 minutes, stirring frequently, then slowly pour in the coconut liquid. Bring to the boil, reduce the heat and simmer for 20 minutes or until the turkey is thoroughly cooked. Stir occasionally during cooking. Mix in the coriander, garnish with coriander sprigs and serve with a large side salad.

## FRUITY CHICKEN SALAD

Preparation time: 15 minutes
Cooking time: 10 minutes
Serves 2

2 chicken breasts
1 tablespoon hot chilli sauce
1 small red onion, thinly sliced
6 radishes, thinly sliced
small bag of mixed baby salad leaves
4 sliced strawberries

For the dressing:
2 tablespoons red wine vinegar
4 tablespoons extra-virgin olive oil
2 strawberries (mashed)

Coat the chicken breasts with the chilli sauce and grill for
10 minutes until thoroughly cooked through, turning
once. Cut into slices and set aside. Toss the rest of the
ingredients together and add the chicken. Combine the
dressing ingredients, then spoon it over the chicken salad.

## TARRAGON TURKEY STEAKS
Preparation time: 30 minutes
Cooking time: 12 minutes
Serves 4

4 large turkey breast steaks
fresh tarragon sprigs, to garnish (optional)
Cauliflower Mash and green beans, to serve

For the marinade:
1 tablespoon Dijon mustard
1 tablespoon orange zest
75ml orange juice
2 tablespoons extra-virgin olive oil
1 tablespoon white wine vinegar
2 tablespoons chopped fresh tarragon

Place the turkey steaks in a shallow dish. Blend the
marinade ingredients, pour over the turkey steaks, cover
and leave to marinate in the fridge for at least 30 minutes
– longer if time permits. Occasionally turn the steaks and
spoon over the marinade. When ready to cook, drain the
turkey, reserving the marinade, and place under a
medium-hot grill. Cook for 10–12 minutes or until
thoroughly cooked, turning at least once and brushing
with the reserved marinade from time to time. Garnish
with the tarragon sprigs, and serve with Cauliflower Mash
(page 111) and green beans.

# CINNAMON DUCK WITH RASPBERRY VINAIGRETTE

Preparation time: 20 minutes
Cooking time: 20 minutes
Serves 2

2 x 175g duck breasts
1 teaspoon ground cinnamon
2 teaspoons sesame seeds
125g fresh raspberries
1 tablespoon balsamic vinegar
2 teaspoons extra-virgin olive oil
freshly ground black pepper
petit pois and new potatoes, to serve

First prepare the vinaigrette. Blend the raspberries in a processor. Then pass the raspberry purée through a sieve and discard the seeds. In a small bowl, whisk together the raspberry purée, vinegar and oil. Season and set aside. Place a frying pan on the heat. Then score the skin side of the duck breasts and sprinkle the skin with cinnamon. Pan-fry the duck, skin side down, until crisp and golden. Turn and continue to cook for 7–9 minutes until cooked through. One minute before the duck is cooked, scatter over the sesame seeds. Remove the duck from the pan and set aside to rest. Slice each duck breast on the diagonal. Drizzle the duck and plate with the raspberry vinaigrette. Serve with petit pois and a few new potatoes.

## CHICKEN PIRI PIRI
Preparation time: 10 minutes
Cooking time: 20 minutes
Serves 4

4 chicken breasts
mixed salad leaves, to serve

For the marinade:
2 tablespoons hot smoked paprika (normal will do)
1 tablespoon minced chilli (or chilli flakes or powder)
1 tablespoon minced garlic
½ handful chopped oregano leaves
½ handful chopped parsley leaves
¼ handful chopped thyme leaves
2 bay leaves, chopped
juice and zest of 2 lemons
3 tablespoons extra-virgin olive oil
freshly ground black pepper

Rub the chicken with the paprika and transfer to a non-metallic bowl. Then add the rest of the marinade ingredients and rub them well into the chicken. Leave it to marinate in the fridge overnight. Bring the chicken to room temperature before lifting it out of its marinade. Then either grill or fry it in a little of the marinade until succulent and cooked through. Serve with mixed salad leaves.

# Fish and shellfish meals

## TUNA STEAKS WITH WILD ROCKET SALSA
Preparation time: 10 minutes
Cooking time: 5 minutes
Serves 4

4 tuna steaks
2 tablespoons chopped fresh dill
½ large cucumber, finely diced
3 tablespoons extra-virgin olive oil
1 tablespoon red wine vinegar
50g wild rocket

Toss the diced cucumber with the wild rocket and dill. Brush the tuna steaks with a bit of the oil and fry for 2–3 minutes each side until just cooked, then remove from the pan. Top each steak with a handful of the wild rocket salsa. Mix the rest of the oil with the vinegar and season. With the pan still on the heat, pour in the vinegar and oil mixture, and sizzle for a few seconds. Then pour it over the tuna and salsa.

# COD WITH CHEDDAR AND CRÈME FRAÎCHE SAUCE

Preparation time: 10 minutes
Cooking time: 20 minutes
Serves 4

4 cod fillets (or any white fish)
225g cherry tomatoes, halved
150g crème fraîche
1 tablespoon wholegrain mustard
freshly ground black pepper
175g half-fat Cheddar cheese, grated

Preheat the oven to 200°C/400°F/Gas Mark 6. Place the cod in a baking dish along with the cherry tomatoes. Combine the crème fraîche and mustard, season and pour over the fish and tomatoes. Sprinkle over the cheese and bake for 20 minutes until the cheese is melted and golden, and the fish is no longer opaque. Serve with low-GL vegetables from the food list in Chapter 4.

# FRESH SPINACH SALMON

Preparation time: 10 minutes
Cooking time: 10 minutes
Serves 2

2 x 200g fresh salmon fillets
1 tablespoon extra-virgin olive oil
1 small onion, finely chopped
100g sliced mushrooms
2 handfuls fresh spinach
grated zest and juice of ½ lemon
freshly ground black pepper
low-GL vegetables, to serve

Season the fish and fry in olive oil for 5 minutes each side, or until cooked through. Set aside and keep warm. Add extra olive oil to the pan and fry the onion. Then add the mushrooms and keep stirring while you add the spinach, cooking it until it wilts. Stir in the lemon zest and juice, and spoon over the fish. Serve with low-GL vegetables.

## NORMANDY-STYLE FISH

Preparation time: 10 minutes
Cooking time: 20 minutes
Serves 2

4 fillets of any white fish
juice of 1 lemon
handful peeled prawns
6 button mushrooms, sliced and fried in olive oil
100ml crème fraîche
1 egg yolk
freshly ground black pepper
salad or low-GL vegetables, to serve

Poach the fish in water for 6–7 minutes until cooked through and no longer opaque, then drain well. Mix the cooked mushrooms, prawns, crème fraîche, lemon juice and pepper, and heat gently for 4 minutes. Remove from the heat and rapidly stir in the egg yolk. Pour over the cooked fish and serve with salad or any low-GL vegetables.

# SALMON WITH CORIANDER PESTO

Preparation time: 10 minutes
Cooking time: 10 minutes
Serves 4

4 fresh salmon fillets
green beans or broccoli and carrots, to serve

For the pesto:
handful chopped coriander
1 clove garlic, crushed
juice of 1 lime plus grated zest
1 red chilli pepper, deseeded and finely chopped
2 tablespoons extra-virgin olive oil
freshly ground black pepper

Place the garlic, coriander, chilli, lime juice and zest, and
a seasoning of black pepper in a food processor. Continue
processing until well chopped and in the meantime pour
in the olive oil to form a wet paste. Preheat the grill to a
high heat and place the salmon on a baking sheet,
spreading the pesto paste on one side of the fish. Cook for
approximately 10 minutes until cooked through. Serve
with green beans or broccoli and carrots.

# FRESH TUNA WITH GARLIC

Preparation time: 10 minutes
Cooking time: 20 minutes
Serves 2

2 fresh tuna steaks
1 tablespoon extra-virgin olive oil
2 tablespoons red wine vinegar
2 cloves garlic (or 1 teaspoon garlic powder)
freshly ground black pepper
salad or Cauli Mash and green beans, to serve

Finely chop the garlic and fry in the olive oil. Season the tuna steaks, add to the pan and fry until cooked through. Remove the steaks and add the red wine vinegar. Reduce to thicken and then pour over the tuna steaks. Serve with salad or Cauliflower Mash (see page 111) and green beans.

## SALMON KEBABS

Preparation time: 10 minutes
Cooking time: 5 minutes
Serves 4

500g fresh salmon, cut into cubes
1 tablespoon chopped fresh mint
2 tablespoons chopped fresh tarragon
3 tablespoons white wine vinegar
freshly ground black pepper
salad or low-GL vegetables, to serve

Mix together the mint, tarragon and vinegar to make a
dressing, seasoning with black pepper to taste. Brush the
salmon liberally with the dressing and grill or barbecue for
5 minutes or until cooked through, turning frequently.
Serve with salad or low-GL vegetables.

# ROAST FISH WITH MUSHROOM AND CORIANDER

Preparation time: 15 minutes
Cooking time: 15 minutes
Serves 4

4 fillets of fish (plaice, cod or any white fish)
80g butter or olive-oil-based spread
1 tablespoon white wine vinegar
12 button mushrooms, finely chopped
100ml crème fraîche
juice of 1 lemon
handful chopped fresh coriander
freshly ground black pepper
asparagus or broccoli, to serve

Preheat the oven to 200°C/400°F/Gas Mark 6. Grease a large ovenproof dish with 50g of the butter or olive-oil-based spread. Make cuts in the fish fillets, place in the dish, and add the lemon juice, white wine vinegar and a seasoning of black pepper. Cook for 15 minutes, basting regularly. Meanwhile, melt the remaining 30g of the butter or olive-oil-based spread in a large pan, add the mushrooms and fry until golden brown. Stir in the coriander and crème fraîche, and heat through. Remove the fish from the oven and pour over the sauce. Serve with low-GL green vegetables such as asparagus or broccoli.

# SALMON AND PRAWN SPAGHETTI

Preparation time: 10 minutes
Cooking time: 20 minutes
Serves 4

4 salmon fillets
400g spaghetti
2 tablespoons cooked peas
125g pack cooked peeled prawns
200ml tub crème fraîche
150ml milk
grated zest and juice of 1 lemon
1 teaspoon grated Parmesan cheese
4–6 basil leaves, torn
freshly ground black pepper

Cook the spaghetti in boiling water until al dente.
Meanwhile, cook the salmon under a preheated hot grill
for 8 minutes, or until just cooked. Flake the salmon flesh
into a bowl, discarding any skin and bones. Drain the
spaghetti and add the salmon, peas, prawns, crème fraîche,
milk, lemon zest and juice. Stir together and heat through.
Stir in the Parmesan, basil leaves and a seasoning of black
pepper, and serve immediately.

## TROUT WITH LEMON AND PINE NUTS

Preparation time: 5 minutes
Cooking time: 5–10 minutes
Serves 2

2 trout fillets
1 garlic clove, finely chopped
50g pine nuts
40g olive-oil-based spread or butter
juice of 1 lemon
salad, to serve

Heat the butter or olive-oil-based spread in a frying pan
and sauté the fish. Add the garlic, pine nuts and lemon
juice, continue to cook the fish for 3–4 minutes each side,
until cooked right through. Serve with a large salad.

## PRAWNS WITH GINGER AND SESAME IN TOMATO SHELLS

Preparation time: 20 minutes
Cooking time: 10 minutes
Serves 2

2 large beef tomatoes
16 uncooked tiger prawns, peeled
1–2 tablespoons sesame oil
2 cloves garlic, very finely sliced
2.5cm piece fresh ginger root, grated (or 1 teaspoon
    ground ginger)
freshly ground black pepper
large salad, to serve

Cut the tomatoes in half and cut a thin slice off the bottom of each half so that it can stand up on a plate. Scoop out the seeds and discard. Heat the sesame oil in a small wok and stir-fry the prawns, garlic and ginger over a gentle heat until the prawns are cooked and have turned pink. Season to taste. Pile the prawns into the tomato shells and drizzle with the pan juices. Serve immediately with the salad.

## CHEESE BAKED COD

Preparation time: 10 minutes
Cooking time: 20 minutes
Serves 2

2 large boneless fillets of cod (or any white fish)
50g half-fat Edam cheese, grated
½ bunch chives, snipped into small pieces
1 heaped teaspoon Dijon mustard
sweetcorn and peas, to serve

Mix together the cheese, chives and mustard to form a paste. Carefully spread the paste over the cod and place it under a hot grill. Cook until the fish is no longer opaque and is thoroughly baked, and the cheese has melted. Serve with low-GL vegetables such as sweetcorn and peas.

## PAN-FRIED SALMON WITH BALSAMIC VINEGAR

Preparation time: 20 minutes
Cooking time: 20 minutes
Serves 4

4 x 175g salmon fillets
450g spinach
25g butter or olive-oil-based spread
drizzle of extra-virgin olive oil

For the dressing:
100ml balsamic vinegar
1 teaspoon Worcestershire sauce
juice of ½ lime or lemon
100ml extra-virgin olive oil
freshly ground black pepper

To prepare the dressing, put the balsamic vinegar and
Worcestershire sauce in a mixing bowl. Stirring constantly
with a wooden spoon, add the lemon or lime juice and
then slowly add the olive oil. Season to taste.

Heat a frying pan until very hot, then add the salmon,
skin side down, and fry for 4–5 minutes, until nearly
cooked through. Turn the salmon over and cook for a
further 3 minutes. Remove from heat, cover and keep
warm. Wash the spinach and place in a large saucepan
with just the water on its leaves. Cook over a gentle heat
until wilted, then drain, squeezing out excess liquid.
Return to the pan, add the butter or olive-oil-based spread
and oil, and stir until the butter has melted and the
spinach is creamy. Season well to taste. Divide the spinach

between four warmed serving plates. Place the salmon on top and spoon 3 tablespoons of balsamic dressing over each piece. Serve immediately with low-GL vegetables from the food list in Chapter 4.

## CANTONESE-STYLE FISH

Preparation time: 10 minutes
Cooking time: 20 minutes
Serves 2

450g firm white fish fillets, such as cod, sole or a whole
    fish such as Dover sole or turbot
1½ tablespoons finely shredded fresh ginger root
    (or 1 teaspoon powdered ginger)
3 tablespoons finely shredded spring onions
2 tablespoons light soy sauce
2 tablespoons dark soy sauce
1 tablespoon groundnut oil
2 teaspoons sesame oil
fresh coriander sprigs, to garnish
low-GL vegetables, to serve

Place the fish on a heatproof plate, scatter it with the
ginger, then steam it until just cooked (it should turn
opaque). Flat fish fillets will take about 5 minutes; whole
fish will take 12–14 minutes. Remove the cooked fish and
pour off the liquid. Scatter it with the spring onions, then
drizzle over the soy sauces. Heat the two oils together in a
small saucepan until smoking, then immediately pour
them over the fish. Garnish with coriander and serve at
once with low-GL vegetables.

# Beef and pork meals

## AVOCADO, BACON AND EGG SALAD
Preparation time: 5 minutes
Cooking time: 10 minutes
Serves 2

1 small bag baby salad leaves
4 eggs
6 slices of lean bacon
1 avocado, destoned and cubed
1 small red onion, finely chopped

Grill the bacon until crispy, then cut into pieces. Boil the eggs until hard-boiled, then cut into quarters. Combine with the remaining ingredients and drizzle with your choice of dressing (see pages 154–55).

## CABBAGE AND HAM BAKE

Preparation time: 10 minutes
Cooking time: 20 minutes
Serves 2

1 medium cabbage, finely shredded and chopped
225g ham, chopped
1 medium onion, finely chopped
175g half-fat Edam cheese, grated
1 teaspoon butter or olive-oil-based spread

Lightly fry the cabbage, onion and ham in the butter/olive oil spread. Transfer to an ovenproof dish and sprinkle with the cheese. Bake in a preheated medium oven for 20 minutes.

## PORK AND RED PEPPER STIR-FRY

Preparation time: 15 minutes
Cooking time: 10 minutes
Serves 2

2 pork fillets, diced*
1 tablespoon extra-virgin olive oil
½ medium onion, chopped
1 red pepper, chopped
1 tablespoon tomato purée
2 tablespoons water
½ teaspoon chilli powder
1 tablespoon single cream or crème fraîche
freshly ground black pepper
mixed salad or low-GL vegetables, to serve

Fry the pork, onion and chilli powder in the olive oil until browned and cooked through. Add the red pepper and cook until softened. Then add all the other ingredients except the cream, stirring continually. Once you have achieved the desired consistency, add the cream and stir again. Serve with a mixed salad or low-GL vegetables.

*Beef, chicken or turkey can also be used instead of pork, if preferred.*

## CABBAGE AND LEEK WITH BACON PESTO

Preparation time: 10 minutes
Cooking time: 20 minutes
Serves 2 as a side dish

½ cabbage
2 large leeks
8 slices lean bacon, chopped
1 tablespoon extra-virgin olive oil
1 clove garlic, crushed
1 small onion, chopped
2 tablespoons red or green pesto
400g tin chopped tomatoes
12 pitted black olives, halved
fresh basil leaves, roughly torn
grated Parmesan (optional)

Heat the oil and add the garlic, onion and bacon. Fry for
6 minutes, stirring occasionally, until cooked through.
Add the pesto, tomatoes and olives and simmer for 2–3
minutes. Meanwhile, slice thinly and steam or boil the
cabbage and leeks for no more than 3–4 minutes. Drain
the vegetables and add to the sauce together with the basil
leaves. Mix together and serve sprinkled with grated
Parmesan as a tasty vegetable side dish.

## STEAK AU POIVRE
Preparation time: 5 minutes
Cooking time: variable
Serves 1

175–275g steak
1 teaspoon black pepper
1 tablespoon cream or 2 tablespoons crème fraîche
2 teaspoons butter or olive-oil-based spread
salad or low-GL green vegetables and new potatoes,
    to serve

Sprinkle the steak with black pepper, then fry it on both
sides in the butter or olive-oil-based spread until cooked to
your preference. Add the cream/crème fraîche to the pan.
Turn the steak over and serve when the cream has heated
through. Serve with a large salad or low-GL green
vegetables and a few new potatoes.

## SAUSAGE AND BACON OMELETTE

Preparation time: 5 minutes
Cooking time: 10 minutes
Serves 2

3 rashers lean bacon, chopped into bits
4 eggs
2 lean, high-meat content sausages
2 large mushrooms, sliced
2 tablespoons butter or olive-oil-based spread
freshly ground black pepper
salad, to serve

Grill the sausages, then cut into chunks. Heat the butter or olive-oil-based spread in a pan and fry the chopped bacon and sausages. Once the bacon is cooked, add the mushrooms and cook for approximately 4 minutes until browned. Beat the eggs, adding black pepper to taste, and pour the omelette mixture into the pan. Tip the pan to ensure all ingredients are well covered, and the omelette is evenly cooked. Once the bottom of the omelette is brown, gently fold over and continue to cook until cooked right through. Remove from the heat and slide on to a plate. Slice and serve with salad. This also makes a delicious weekend or 'treat' breakfast.

## SPICED BEEF WITH APRICOTS

Preparation time: 10 minutes
Cooking time: 15 minutes
Serves 2

225g lean minced or cubed beef
1 tablespoon extra-virgin olive oil
2 leeks, chopped
3 garlic cloves, finely chopped
1 medium onion, thinly sliced
4 fresh apricots, peeled, pitted and chopped
1 cinnamon stick
2 teaspoons finely chopped ginger root
2 teaspoons grated orange rind
juice of 2 oranges
freshly ground black pepper

Heat the olive oil in a pan, add the onion, garlic and
cinnamon, and fry gently until brown. Add the minced
beef and cook gently, stirring constantly for 5 minutes.
When the meat is browned and cooked through, add the
apricots, ginger, leeks, and orange juice and rind. Cover
and cook for a further 8–10 minutes until all the
vegetables are soft. Season with black pepper, then remove
the cinnamon stick. Serve with low-GL vegetables from
the food list in Chapter 4.

## SWEET AND SOUR PORK

Preparation time: 10 minutes
Cooking time: 12 minutes
Serves 2

250g lean pork fillet, thinly sliced
3 tablespoons extra-virgin olive oil
1 garlic clove, finely chopped
1 small red pepper and yellow pepper, deseeded and
    finely sliced
4 spring onions, chopped into 4cm lengths
10ml white wine vinegar
50ml water
1 tablespoon soy sauce
½ teaspoon fructose
1 teaspoon tomato purée
1 spring onion, finely chopped, to garnish
low-GL vegetables, to serve

Heat 2 tablespoons of the olive oil in a pan and stir-fry the
pork over a medium heat for 5 minutes. Remove and set
aside. Heat the remaining olive oil in the pan and sauté
the garlic, peppers and spring onions for 3 minutes. Return
the pork to the pan, stir in the fructose, white wine
vinegar, water, tomato purée and soy sauce, and simmer for
3 minutes. Garnish with finely chopped spring onion and
serve with low-GL vegetables.

## ROSEMARY PORK TENDERLOIN

Preparation: 2 hours
Cooking time: 20 minutes
Serves 2


2 pork tenderloins*
low-GL vegetables, to serve

For the marinade:
4 tablespoons extra-virgin olive oil
1 tablespoon minced garlic
2 tablespoons chopped fresh rosemary
½ teaspoon black pepper


Blend the marinade ingredients, pour over the pork and leave it to soak in the fridge for 2 hours. Place the pork under a hot grill with a little of its marinade until thoroughly cooked, making sure the meat is no longer pink in the centre. Serve with low-GL roast vegetables.

* *This recipe also works well with lamb*

## VENETIAN LIVER

Preparation time: 20 minutes
Cooking time: 10 minutes
Serves 2

200g liver, cut into shreds
1 tablespoon extra-virgin olive oil
1 sweet potato, peeled and cubed
125g broccoli, shredded
¼ teaspoon cumin seeds
¼ teaspoon coriander seeds
2 tablespoons red wine
1 tablespoon snipped fresh chives
low-GL vegetables, to serve

In a medium sauté pan, dry-fry the spices to release the oil and flavour, then stir in the oil and heat. Fry the potatoes until lightly browned. Add the liver and cook for 2 minutes. Stir in the broccoli and cook for a further 2 minutes. Pour in the wine and simmer for 1 minute. Fold through the chives and serve with low-GL vegetables.

## MARINATED BEEF STRIPS

Preparation time: 1 hour
Cooking time: 10 minutes
Serves 4

500g lean tender beefsteak, cut against the grain into 8 x
5cm rectangles
5 medium mushrooms, thinly sliced
125g onions, peeled and sliced thickly
3 spring onions, cut into 5cm chunks
1 medium carrot, peeled and cut into 5cm chunks, then
    cut lengthways into slices
2 tablespoons sesame oil
1 tablespoon roasted sesame seeds
1 dessertspoon fructose

For the marinade:
½ medium-sized hard pear, peeled, cored and chopped
4 garlic cloves, peeled and chopped
5cm cube fresh ginger root, peeled and chopped
    (or 1 teaspoon ground ginger)
4 tablespoons soy sauce

Mix the pear, garlic, ginger and soy sauce in a blender until
smooth. Place the meat in a bowl and add the paste from
the blender, together with the mushrooms, onions, spring
onions, carrot, sesame oil, sesame seeds and fructose. Mix
well, cover and marinate for 1–2 hours. Set a large heavy
frying pan on a high heat until very hot. Fry the meat layer
by layer, then add the vegetables and marinade. Cook on a
high heat for a few minutes. Spoon the mixture over the
meat. Serve with low-GL vegetables.

# BEEF CURRY

Preparation time: 20 minutes
Cooking time: 20 minutes
Serves 2

300g sirloin steak, cubed*
2 tablespoons extra-virgin olive oil
½ onion, peeled and finely chopped
2 garlic cloves, peeled and finely chopped
200g sweet potatoes, cut into 2.5cm cubes
2 teaspoons tomato purée
4 plum tomatoes, diced
¼ teaspoon ground turmeric
¼ teaspoon ground ginger (or 2.5cm piece fresh ginger
    root, grated)
1 teaspoon medium curry powder
2 teaspoons chopped fresh thyme leaves
¼ teaspoon crushed dried chilli flakes
¼ teaspoon coriander seeds
3 cardamom pods, lightly crushed
150ml beef stock
2 teaspoons chopped fresh mint
1 tablespoon chopped fresh coriander
freshly ground black pepper

In a frying pan, dry-fry the turmeric, ginger, curry powder,
chilli flakes, coriander seeds and cardamom pods for 1
minute. Then heat the olive oil in a medium sauté pan.
Season the steak and fry it for 2–3 minutes. Add the onion
and cook for 1–2 minutes until softened. Stir in the garlic,
dry-fried spices, thyme, potatoes and tomato purée. Pour

in the stock, bring to a simmering point and cook for 10 minutes. Add the tomatoes and cook for a further 3 minutes. Fold in the mint and coriander, and serve.

* *This recipe also works well with lamb*

# PEPPERED PORK WITH CHESTNUT MUSHROOMS
Preparation time: 10 minutes
Cooking time: 30 minutes
Serves 2

2 x 175g pork fillets
2 tablespoons crushed black peppercorns
10 chestnut mushrooms
10 asparagus tips
2 shallots, chopped
1 clove garlic, chopped
2 tablespoons French mustard
4 tablespoons double cream/crème fraîche
knob of butter

Roll the pork fillets in the crushed peppercorns until fully coated. Then put the pork in a roasting tray and drizzle with a little olive oil. Place on the middle shelf of the oven at 220°C/425°F/Gas Mark 7 for about 15–20 minutes, turning once halfway through. Trim the asparagus to about 5cm long and cook in boiling water for 3 minutes. Then place them in cold water and set aside. Melt a little butter in a saucepan and sweat the shallots on a low to medium heat for about 4–5 minutes. Add the garlic and mushrooms and cook for 4 minutes, then add the asparagus, cream/crème fraîche and mustard. Reduce the sauce by about a third. When the pork is cooked, place in the centre of a plate, spoon the sauce around and arrange the vegetables on the side. Serve immediately.

## ROASTED PEANUT-CRUSTED PORK CHOPS

Preparation time: 20 minutes
Cooking time: 15 minutes
Serves 2

4 pork chops
3 tablespoons extra-virgin olive oil
340g chunky, sugar-free peanut butter (we love the Whole
    Earth organic variety)
4 tablespoons tomato purée
4 tablespoons lime juice
1 onion, finely chopped
3 garlic cloves, crushed
1 teaspoon paprika
½ teaspoon mixed spice
2.5cm piece fresh ginger root, grated (or 1 teaspoon
    ground ginger)
low-GL vegetables, to serve

Mix all the ingredients together into a smooth paste and
marinate the pork chops for about 30 minutes. Set the
oven to 190°C/375°F/Gas Mark 5. Arrange the pork and
marinade on an oiled baking tray and cover with foil.
Cook both sides for about 10 minutes, adding 5 extra
minutes to be sure it's completely done. Serve with low-
GL vegetables.

## Vegetarian Meals and Side Dishes

MOZZARELLA, TOMATO AND ASPARAGUS SALAD
Preparation time: 10 minutes
Cooking time: 4 minutes
Serves 4

175g mozzarella cheese, cut into cubes
fresh asparagus (4–5 spears per person)
16 cherry tomatoes, halved
4 fresh basil leaves

Cook the asparagus in boiling water for about 4 minutes until slightly softened. Drain and put in cold water to cool. Mix the asparagus with the cherry tomatoes and mozzarella. Add a dressing of your choice (see pages 154–55) and decorate with torn basil leaves.

## COUSCOUS SALAD

Preparation time: 15 minutes
Cooking time: 15–30 minutes
Serves 6

150g couscous
2 tablespoons of extra-virgin olive oil
2 large tomatoes
2 large or 4 small onions (or 6 spring onions),
    finely chopped
2 tablespoons of harissa paste (hot red pepper paste)
juice and zest of 1 lemon
a large bunch of parsley, finely chopped
handful fresh mint, finely chopped
fresh lemon wedges and dips, to serve

Cook the couscous as per the packet instructions. While it is cooking, blanch the tomatoes in boiling water for 1 minute, remove and peel. Cut open, discard the wet insides and chop the rest finely. Once the couscous is cooked, mix in all the ingredients, including the hot paste. Serve with fresh lemon wedges on the side and a selection of the dips from pages 156–58.

## WILD MUSHROOM AND PEARL BARLEY 'RISOTTO'

Preparation time: 10 minutes
Cooking time: 35–40 minutes
Serves 4

150g wild mushrooms (chanterelle, shiitake, button, ceps,
    oyster), roughly sliced
120g pearl barley
25g butter or olive-oil-based spread
1 teaspoon extra-virgin olive oil
2 cloves of garlic, finely chopped
1 medium onion/3 shallots, finely chopped
100ml dry white wine
700ml chicken stock
handful chopped fresh herbs (basil, parsley and
    coriander), to garnish
25g Parmesan, shaved or grated (or Mature Cheddar),
    to garnish
asparagus spears, to serve

Using a large frying pan, melt half the butter or olive-oil-
based spread and the olive oil on a medium heat, add the
mushrooms and cook for about 3–4 minutes, until lightly
browned. Put into a bowl and set aside. On a moderate
heat, melt the rest of the butter spread and fry the onions
for about a minute, stirring gently. Then add the garlic and
cook for a further 2–3 minutes – don't let the garlic burn.
Pour in the wine to deglaze the pan and get all the flavour
from the bottom, increase the heat and bring to the boil,
stirring constantly. Boil for 4–5 minutes, stirring until it
reaches a syrupy thickness. Turn down the heat and add

the barley and mushrooms, stirring them together well. Add about a third of the chicken stock and, stirring constantly, cook until all the liquid has been absorbed by the barley. Continue adding liquid until it has been completely absorbed – it should take about 35–40 minutes. Serve with steamed asparagus spears, with chopped fresh herbs and Parmesan scattered on top.

# WATERMELON, MINT AND FETA SALAD
Preparation time: 10 minutes
Serves 2–3

½ watermelon
1 packet of feta, cut into small cubes
handful fresh mint, roughly chopped
juice of ½ lemon

Chop the watermelon into chunks, discarding the seeds, and put it in a large salad bowl. Sprinkle it with the cubed feta, followed by the chopped mint. Then squeeze the lemon juice over the salad, toss and serve.

## GARLIC MUSHROOMS WITH CHEESE
Preparation time: 10 minutes
Cooking time: 6 minutes
Serves 2 as a main course, 4 as a starter

2 medium packs of any mushrooms (oyster, shiitake,
   chestnut, button or a combination)
2 cloves garlic, finely chopped
1 teaspoon red chilli flakes (or fresh chilli)
1 tablespoon butter
1 tablespoon extra-virgin olive oil
1 teaspoon grain mustard
handful chopped chives
Manchego (Spanish ewe's cheese) or Parmesan,
   to garnish

Rinse the mushrooms quickly and drain. Warm a large frying pan on a medium heat, add the butter and the olive oil, and allow to melt. Add the garlic, chilli flakes and the mustard, and allow to infuse in the warming oil. When ready, throw in the mushrooms and toss them in the mixture, allowing them to warm through for about 6–8 minutes. Shave some Manchego or Parmesan over each plate, sprinkle with chives and serve.

## ROASTED VEGETABLES
Preparation time: 20 minutes
Cooking time: 40 minutes
Serves 6

1 medium celeriac, cleaned, peeled and cut into chunks
(about 5cm square)
4 carrots, washed, peeled if necessary and cut into chunks
½ swede, washed, peeled and cut into chunks
1 medium-size sweet potato, washed, peeled and cut into
   chunks
2 large red onions, peeled and cut into quarters
1 bulb garlic, cloves separated but left in skins
4 sprigs fresh rosemary
60ml (approx) extra-virgin olive oil

Half fill a large pan with boiling water and carefully add all
the vegetables, except the onion and garlic, plus more water
to cover if necessary. In the meantime pour the olive oil on
to a large baking tray (enough to cover the bottom) and put
it in a preheated oven (200°C/400°F/Gas Mark 6). Boil the
vegetables rapidly for about 5–7 minutes, drain, then put
them back in the pan. Put on the lid and hold it down while
you shake the pan about to 'bash' the vegetables a little.
Carefully take the now-hot baking tray out of the oven and
transfer the vegetables on to the tray, along with the onions.
Try to make sure all the vegetables have a coating of oil.
Place the whole garlic cloves around the tray and lay the
rosemary sprigs in between the vegetables. Put back in the
oven, and roast for approximately 40 minutes, turning and
basting halfway through.

## GREEN BEAN FRITTATA

Preparation time: 10 minutes
Cooking time: 20 minutes
Serves 2

250g runner beans, sliced
250g peas
1 tablespoon extra-virgin olive oil
30g butter or olive-oil-based spread
50g Gruyère cheese (or similar), grated
2 tablespoons chopped chives
6 eggs
freshly ground black pepper
salad, to serve

Cook the beans and peas in salted boiling water until tender, then drain. Beat the eggs with black pepper. Stir in the chives, beans and peas. Heat the butter or olive-oil-based spread and oil in a large frying pan. Add the egg and vegetable mixture, and spread evenly in the pan. Cook on a low heat for 10 minutes until golden brown. Sprinkle with the grated cheese and grill for 2 minutes until the cheese has melted. Serve hot or cold, sliced into wedges with salad.

## VEGETARIAN SAUSAGE AND SWEET POTATO MASH

Preparation time: 15 minutes
Cooking time: 20 minutes
Serves 2

2 medium sweet potatoes*
1 medium onion, finely chopped
1 tablespoon extra-virgin olive oil
6 Quorn or soya sausages
peas and green beans, to serve

Peel and boil the potatoes until tender, or bake in their skins in the microwave until soft inside and then peel away the skin. Meanwhile, grill the sausages until cooked through. Mash the sweet potato, then fry the onions in olive oil until browned. Arrange on a plate and serve with peas and green beans.

*Although sweet potatoes have a lower GL than ordinary white potatoes, they are still medium GL so have them only occasionally. Another good tip is to combine them with another vegetable (carrots, celeriac or cauliflower) as a mash – not only delicious but lower GL.

## VEGETARIAN STUFFED AUBERGINE

Preparation time: 15 minutes
Cooking time: 45 minutes
Serves 2

250g soya mince
1 aubergine cut in half lengthwise
1 tablespoon extra-virgin olive oil
225g feta cheese, cubed
200g tin chopped tomatoes
225g frozen chopped spinach
1 onion, finely chopped
2 cloves garlic, finely chopped (or ½ teaspoon garlic
  powder)
2 teaspoons oregano
juice of 1 lemon
freshly ground black pepper

Preheat the oven to a high heat. Put the two halves of aubergine, cut side down, on a baking sheet sprayed with olive oil. Bake for 25 minutes, or until very tender, and set aside to cool – leave the oven on. While the aubergine is baking, fry the soya with the garlic, onions and seasonings in olive oil for 4–5 minutes – add water if the mixture appears dry. Add the tomatoes, spinach and lemon juice, simmer and stir for 5 minutes. Scoop out the flesh of the aubergine, chop and add to the soya mixture. Scoop the mixture back into aubergine halves, then bake in the oven for 15 minutes. Top with crumbled feta cheese and bake for an extra 5 minutes. Serve with salad or low-GL vegetables.

# CAULIFLOWER MASH

Preparation time: 10 minutes
Cooking time: 10 minutes
Serves 2

1 medium-sized cauliflower, cut into quarters and green
    leaves removed
100g grated half-fat Edam or similar
2 teaspoons butter- or olive-oil-based spread
small amount of crème fraîche, cream or milk (optional)
1 teaspoon mustard (optional)
freshly ground black pepper

Boil or steam the cauliflower, then drain very thoroughly
so it is as dry as possible. Blend it in a food processor until
smooth. Add the rest of the ingredients and a twist of
black pepper, being careful to add liquids very gradually
and stop when you have the right consistency – don't add
too much liquid. You could also add a small amount of
Parmesan or other cheese with a strong flavour instead of
the Edam. Reheat and serve as you would mashed potato.

*Note: Cauliflower has a very low GL compared with normal
white potatoes and is a healthy alternative to mashed potato. It
makes a delicious topping for shepherd's pie and fish pie. Just
place on top of the pie mixture, sprinkle with grated cheese and
cook in the oven until the cheese has melted and turned golden
brown on top. This recipe also works well with other lower-GL
root vegetables, such as carrots, celeriac, swede, and so on.
Mash them with the cauliflower, or alone, or have a
combination of them all.*

## VEGETABLE KEBABS

Preparation time: 15 minutes
Cooking time: 15 minutes
Serves 2

8 cherry tomatoes
8 button mushrooms
8 shallots
1 red and 1 yellow pepper with stem and seeds removed,
    cut into quarters
1 tablespoon extra-virgin olive oil
1 teaspoon mixed herbs
freshly ground black pepper
tomato-style sauce, to serve

Thread the vegetables alternately on to 2 large or 4 small
skewers. Brush with olive oil and sprinkle with the pepper
and herbs. Cook under a medium grill, turning frequently
to avoid burning. Serve with a tomato-style sauce.

# SWEET POTATO AND WALNUT SALAD

Preparation time: 20 minutes
Cooking time: 20 minutes
Serves 2

2 large sweet potatoes, peeled and cubed into 2.5cm
    squares
1 tablespoon chopped walnuts
1 tablespoon extra-virgin olive oil
1 tablespoon orange juice (with bits)
1 red apple, sliced
juice of 1 lemon
1 teaspoon chopped fresh parsley
freshly ground black pepper

Boil the potatoes until tender, then drain and leave to
cool down. In the meantime put the rest of the ingredients
in a large bowl and mix them well together. Then add the
potatoes and serve with a baby leaf salad and cherry
tomatoes.

## VEGETARIAN KORMA

Preparation time: 10 minutes
Cooking time: 30 minutes
Serves 4

350g Quorn pieces
3 tablespoons extra-virgin olive oil
50g cashews
60g natural unsweetened yoghurt
4 garlic cloves, crushed (or 2 teaspoons garlic paste)
1 large onion, chopped
2 bay leaves, crumbled
2 teaspoons ground coriander
½ teaspoon chilli powder
½ teaspoon ground cumin
1 small cube of ginger root, peeled and grated (or 1
   teaspoon ground ginger)
½ teaspoon ground turmeric
½ teaspoon paprika
freshly ground black pepper
425ml boiling water
125ml cold water
paprika, to garnish
1 tablespoon toasted flaked almonds, to garnish
salad, to serve

Heat the oil in a heavy-based pan, then add the bay
leaves, onion, garlic and ginger. Fry until the onion turns
golden brown. Next, add the coriander, cumin, turmeric,
chilli and pepper. Fry for 30 seconds. Add 75ml boiling
water and stir until the water evaporates. Then add the

Quorn and fry for 2 minutes. Add half of the yoghurt and 350ml boiling water. Blend the cashews with 125ml cold water in a blender, add the remaining yoghurt, purée until smooth, then add to the pan. Cover and simmer for 15–20 minutes, stirring occasionally. Simmer uncovered to reduce the sauce, if necessary. Transfer to a dish, garnish with the toasted almonds and sprinkle with paprika. Serve with a tossed salad.

## VEGETABLE AND CHICKPEA TAGINE

Preparation time: 10 minutes
Cooking time: 30 minutes
Serves 4

2 x 250g packs of ready-prepared vegetables
400g can chickpeas, drained
400g can chopped tomatoes with garlic
1 tablespoon extra-virgin olive oil
1 red onion, thinly sliced
1 red chilli, chopped
100g dried apricots, chopped
1 teaspoon ground cumin
2 tablespoons chopped fresh coriander

Heat the oil in a large pan and add the onion until softened. Add the cumin and chilli and cook for 1 minute. Add the apricots, vegetables and tomatoes, and stir. Fill the empty tomato can with water and add to the pan, then season and bring to the boil. Lower the heat, cover and simmer for 15 minutes. Add the chickpeas, then cook for a further 10 minutes or until the vegetables are tender. Stir in the coriander and serve.

# LINGUINE WITH BLACK OLIVE PESTO
Preparation time: 20 minutes
Cooking time: 20 minutes
Serves 4

320g fresh linguine pasta or similar
2 tablespoons black olive paste
4 tablespoons extra-virgin olive oil
2 tablespoons pine nut kernels
1 clove garlic, chopped
40g grated Parmesan
juice and zest of 1 lemon (unwaxed)
handful fresh parsley, stalks removed
freshly ground black pepper

Toast the pine nuts gently in a dry frying pan until golden
brown. Transfer to a food processor with the parsley, garlic,
lemon zest and black olive paste. While mixing, drizzle in
enough olive oil to form a thick paste. Transfer to a large
bowl, stir in the Parmesan and season to taste. Cook the
pasta until cooked al dente. Drain and toss with the black
olive pesto. Stir in the lemon juice to taste.

*Black olive pesto also makes a delicious sauce for 'vegetable
pasta' – using shredded vegetables or strips of vegetables instead
of the pasta (and in larger amounts). Boil or steam the
vegetables until cooked al dente, then drain. Toss in the olive
pesto, and stir in lemon juice to taste.*

# GARLIC AND CHILLI CABBAGE AND LEEK

Preparation time: 10 minutes
Cooking time: 10 minutes
Serves 3–4 as a side dish

1 medium-sized cabbage
1 leek per person
1 tablespoon hot chilli flakes or fresh red chilli
   chopped finely
2 cloves garlic, finely chopped
2 tablespoons butter or extra-virgin olive oil

Shred the cabbage, cut the leeks into rings and rinse all in cold water. Using a large enough pan to hold the cabbage and leeks (if you have a steamer, it is preferable to steam the vegetables), fill with enough water to cover, and bring to the boil. Boil for 5 minutes until just cooked – but still with some crunch left. Set a large frying pan on a medium heat, warm the butter/olive oil, and add the garlic and chilli. Drain the vegetables well, then transfer to the frying pan and toss them in the mixture. Serve immediately.

*Purple sprouting broccoli (when available) is a nice alternative to the cabbage and leeks, served with a few shavings of Parmesan over the finished dish.*

## BALTI-STYLE CAULIFLOWER WITH TOMATOES

Preparation time: 10 minutes

Cooking time: 15 minutes

Serves 2

1 cauliflower, broken into florets

4 plum tomatoes, quartered

2 tablespoons extra-virgin olive oil

1 onion, finely chopped

2 garlic cloves, crushed

175g fresh spinach, roughly chopped

175ml water

1–2 tablespoons lemon juice

1 teaspoon ground coriander

1 teaspoon ground cumin

1 teaspoon ground fennel seeds

½ teaspoon garam masala

pinch ground ginger (or 2.5cm piece fresh
    ginger root, grated)

½ teaspoon chilli powder

freshly ground black pepper

soya mince or vegetarian sausages, to serve

Heat the oil in a wok or a large frying pan. Add the onion and garlic and stir-fry for 3 minutes until the onions are browned. Add the cauliflower and stir-fry for a further 3 minutes until flecked with brown. Add the coriander, cumin, fennel seeds, garam masala, ginger and chilli powder, and cook over a high heat for 1 minute, stirring continuously. Add the tomatoes, water and pepper and bring to the boil. Reduce the heat, cover and simmer for 6 minutes until the cauliflower is tender. Stir in the chopped spinach, cover and cook for 1 minute until the spinach is tender. Add enough lemon juice to sharpen the flavour and adjust seasoning to taste. Serve with soya mince or vegetarian sausages.

## BRAISED CELERY WITH GOAT'S CHEESE
Preparation time: 10 minutes
Cooking time: 20 minutes
Serves 2

1 head of celery, thinly sliced
175g goat's cheese
30g butter or olive-oil-based spread
3–4 tablespoons single cream or crème fraîche
freshly ground black pepper
peas and carrots, to serve

Preheat the oven to 180°C/350°F/Gas Mark 4 and lightly
butter a shallow ovenproof dish. Melt the butter or olive-
oil-based spread in a saucepan and fry the celery for 3
minutes, stirring continuously. Add 3–4 tablespoons of
water to the pan, heat gently, then cover and simmer over
a low heat for 6 minutes or until tender. Remove the pan
from the heat and stir in the goat's cheese and
cream/crème fraîche. Season and turn into a prepared
dish. Cover the dish with buttered greaseproof paper and
bake in the preheated oven for 10–12 minutes. Serve with
peas and carrots.

# VEGETABLES WITH GUACAMOLE TOPPING

Preparation time: 15 minutes
Cooking time: 12 minutes
Serves 1

handful broccoli florets
handful cauliflower florets
2–3 carrots, sliced lengthways
1 medium leek, sliced into rings
125g green beans

For the guacamole topping:
½ avocado, mashed
1 spring onion, finely chopped
2 cherry tomatoes
1 teaspoon curry paste
1 teaspoon chopped coriander
¼ teaspoon garlic powder
freshly ground black pepper

Steam the broccoli, carrots, cauliflower, leek and green beans for 10 minutes. Spoon the avocado into a bowl and, using a fork, mix it with the spring onion, curry paste, coriander, tomatoes, garlic and seasoning of pepper. When the vegetables are cooked, drain and serve topped with the guacamole.

## TOMATO AND COURGETTE BAKE

Preparation time: 10 minutes
Cooking time: 40 minutes
Serves 2

2 courgettes, thinly sliced
6 small tomatoes, halved
2 teaspoons extra-virgin olive oil
2 teaspoons chopped thyme
2 garlic cloves, finely chopped
4 eggs
3 tablespoons semi-skimmed milk
2 tablespoons freshly grated Parmesan
freshly ground black pepper
salad, to serve

Oil an ovenproof dish and scatter with the courgettes, garlic, thyme and tomatoes. Season lightly. Add the oil and toss to mix. Bake in a preheated oven (200°C/400°F/Gas Mark 6) for 10 minutes. Lightly beat the eggs with the milk, add pepper and pour the mixture over the vegetables. Sprinkle with the Parmesan and bake for 30 minutes until golden. Serve with a salad.

## BALSAMIC VEGETABLE STIR-FRY

Preparation time: 10 minutes
Cooking time: 10 minutes
Serves 1

75g green beans
125g mushrooms
6 cherry tomatoes, halved
4 spring onions, chopped
handful broccoli florets
handful cauliflower florets
2 rosemary sprigs
1 tablespoon balsamic vinegar
approx 150ml vegetable stock
handful basil leaves, torn into pieces
basil leaves, to serve

Heat the stock with the rosemary sprigs in a large wok or frying pan until it comes to the boil. Chop the beans, broccoli, cauliflower and mushrooms, and add to the boiling stock. Cover the pan and cook for 5 minutes, making sure the vegetables don't stick to the pan. Add the cherry tomatoes, spring onions and balsamic vinegar, and cook for 1 minute, stirring continually. Serve scattered with basil leaves.

## PASTA WITH LENTIL AND RED PEPPER SAUCE

Preparation time: 10 minutes
Cooking time: 30 minutes
Serves 4

320g pasta
250g tin of tomatoes
1 tablespoon tomato purée
100g split red lentils
2 tablespoons extra-virgin olive oil
1 small red pepper, deseeded and chopped
1 medium onion, peeled and chopped
1 clove garlic, crushed
1 teaspoon basil
1 teaspoon butter or olive-oil-based spread
400ml water
2 tablespoons grated cheese
salt and pepper

In a large saucepan, fry the onion and pepper in the oil for
10 minutes. Next, add the garlic, basil, tomatoes, lentils,
tomato purée and water. Bring to the boil, then reduce the
heat to simmer gently uncovered for 15–20 minutes, until
the lentils are cooked. Season with pepper. About 15
minutes before the sauce is ready, half fill a large saucepan
with water and bring to the boil, adding the pasta. Boil
rapidly uncovered for a few minutes until cooked al dente.
Drain, then return to the pan with the butter, and season
with salt and pepper. Dish it up with the sauce and
sprinkle with the grated cheese. Serve with lots of low-GL
vegetables of your choice.

## CURRIED MUSHROOMS

Preparation time: 5 minutes
Cooking time: 25 minutes
Serves 2

250g mushrooms, washed and finely sliced
1 large onion, finely sliced
2 large beef tomatoes
2 tablespoons extra-virgin olive oil
¼ teaspoon turmeric
chilli, to taste
peas and carrots, to serve

Heat the oil in a saucepan, add the turmeric, chilli and onions, and fry until soft. Add the tomatoes and cook for 3 minutes, stirring all the time. Add the mushrooms, cover and simmer for 15–20 minutes. Remove the lid and dry out all the water. Serve hot with peas and carrots.

## TOMATO OMELETTE

Preparation time: 5 minutes
Cooking time: 5 minutes
Serves 2

6 medium tomatoes, cut into slices
4 eggs
2 tablespoons chopped fresh basil
2 tablespoons butter or olive-oil-based spread
freshly ground black pepper
baby leaf salad, cucumber and coleslaw, to serve

Beat the eggs and add the tomato slices, basil and seasoning. Heat the butter or olive-oil-based spread in a frying pan and pour in the omelette mixture. Tip the pan to ensure all the mixture is evenly cooked. Fold the omelette on to a plate. Serve with a baby leaf salad, cucumber and coleslaw.

## QUICK VEGETABLE STIR-FRY

Preparation time: 15 minutes
Cooking time: 10 minutes
Serves 4

500g broccoli, broken into small florets
125g carrots, peeled and cut into matchsticks
125g mangetout
1 red pepper, deseeded and chopped
1 yellow pepper, deseeded and chopped
8 spring onions, trimmed and finely chopped
3 cloves garlic, peeled and grated
2.5cm piece ginger root, grated (or 1 teaspoon
    ground ginger)
3 tablespoons groundnut oil/walnut oil
2 tablespoons vegetable stock or water
1 tablespoon soy sauce
black pepper to taste

Heat the oil in a wok until hot, add the garlic and ginger and stir-fry for 1 minute. Add the broccoli, carrots and peppers, and stir-fry for 5 minutes. Add the stock and mangetout and cook for a further 3 minutes. Stir in the soy sauce, sprinkle over the spring onions, season, stir and serve.

## BROCCOLI AND LEEKS WITH BLUE CHEESE SAUCE

Preparation time: 6 minutes
Cooking time: 12 minutes
Serves 6

480g pasta
400g broccoli florets, separated
2 medium leeks, finely sliced
1½ tablespoons extra-virgin olive oil
150ml vegetable stock
142ml tub single cream or crème fraîche
125g soft blue cheese such as Dolceletta, cubed
75g walnuts, chopped
freshly ground black pepper

Cook the pasta until al dente, adding the broccoli a few minutes before the end of cooking time. In a frying pan, heat the oil and fry the leeks until tender. Season with black pepper. Add the stock, cream and cheese, and cook until the sauce has melted. Stir in the nuts. Drain the pasta and broccoli, stir in the sauce and serve.

## VIETNAMESE COCONUT VEGETABLES

Preparation time: 15 minutes
Cooking time: 25 minutes
Serves 2

1 packet tofu
3 handfuls vegetables (broccoli, cauliflower, carrots,
    green beans, peas)
2 tablespoons olive oil
1 packet creamed coconut
2 tablespoons dark soy sauce
1 tablespoon light soy sauce

Drain the tofu thoroughly (gently press it with a bit of kitchen paper to absorb the moisture). Cut into cubes and fry in hot oil. Set aside. Wash and prepare the vegetables into bite-sized pieces. Set aside. Add enough boiling water to the creamed coconut to make it up to 500ml and stir well. Put this in a wok (with a lid), or a large saucepan. Add the soy sauces and bring to the boil. Now add the tofu and vegetables. Put the lid on tightly and simmer for 20 minutes, or until the vegetables are done. Serve hot.

# CHERRY TOMATO, CHEESE AND RED ONION UPSIDE-DOWN CAKE

Preparation time: 20 minutes
Cooking time: 20 minutes
Serves 4–6 as a side dish


4–6 cherry tomatoes
2 large red onions, chopped
1 tablespoon olive oil
handful fresh rosemary, washed and chopped finely
1 teaspoon caraway seeds
freshly ground black pepper


For the cake:
50g strong cheese (such as Mature Cheddar or Parmesan)
75g ground almonds
2 large eggs
4 tablespoons (60ml) water
1 teaspoon baking powder
1 teaspoon mustard (optional)


Chop the onions and fry in a tablespoon of olive oil, over a medium heat, until slightly brown. Add the rosemary to the pan, being careful not to burn, then put aside. In the meantime, select two medium-sized mixing bowls. Into one bowl, put the ground almonds, cheese (grated or crumbled), baking powder and water (and mustard, if using). Separate the eggs and add the yolks to the mixture, putting the whites into the other mixing bowl. Whisk the egg whites first, until fluffy and holding their shape. Then whisk the cheese mixture – it should still be quite thick but pourable. Grease a shallow cake tin with olive oil. Arrange the fried onions in the bottom of the tin, place the cherry tomatoes around them at regular intervals, then sprinkle with the caraway seeds and some black pepper. Fold the egg white into the cheese mixture, until combined. Then pour this over the onions and tomatoes in the cake tin. Bake for 15–20 minutes in a preheated oven (190°C/375°F/Gas Mark 5). Remove it from the oven when golden and firm. Allow it to cool slightly, slice and serve. This cake is also delicious when eaten cold.

## CHICKPEA CURRY

Preparation time: 10 minutes
Cooking time: 10 minutes
Serves 1

1 tin chickpeas, drained and rinsed
1 tablespoon olive oil
1 fresh tomato, chopped (or 1 small tin tomatoes)
1 onion, chopped
1 clove garlic, crushed
5cm piece ginger root, grated (or 1 teaspoon ground
    ginger)
¼ teaspoon red chilli powder
½ teaspoon cumin powder
¼ teaspoon coriander powder
¼ teaspoon turmeric
pinch garam masala
low-GL vegetables, to serve

Heat a deep saucepan or a medium-sized wok and add the oil followed by the onions and garlic. Fry the mixture until the onions are caramelised. Then add the cumin, coriander, turmeric and red chilli powders. Mix for 1 minute, then tip in the tomatoes. Cook the sauce until it begins to thicken. Add one cup of water and stir. Then add the chickpeas and mix, mashing a few of the chickpeas while cooking. Cover and simmer for 5 minutes, then add the ginger and garam masala. Cook for another minute. Serve with low-GL vegetables.

# VEGETABLE KEBABS WITH GADO GADO SAUCE

Preparation time: 30 minutes
Cooking time: 30 minutes
Serves 2

1 large aubergine
1 red pepper
1 green pepper
2 courgettes
8 mushrooms
4 tomatoes
3 tablespoons extra-virgin olive oil
1 tablespoon lemon juice
2 tablespoons chopped fresh coriander
freshly ground black pepper

For the sauce:
1 large onion, chopped
2 cloves garlic, crushed
50g butter or olive-oil-based spread
1 red chilli, deseeded and chopped
1 teaspoon grated fresh ginger root (or ½ teaspoon
   ground ginger)
150ml sugar-free peanut butter
1 teaspoon fructose
1 lemon, juice only
300ml water
1 bay leaf
dash soy sauce
dash cider vinegar

Cut the aubergine, peppers and courgettes into 1 inch (5cm) pieces. Halve the mushrooms and tomatoes. Mix the olive oil, lemon juice, coriander and pepper, and marinate all the vegetables. To make the sauce, melt the butter or olive-oil-based spread and sweat the onion and garlic until soft. Then add all the other sauce ingredients and cook on a low heat for 20 minutes. While the sauce is cooking, thread the vegetables on metal skewers. Place them on to a baking sheet and grill until browned, then slide the vegetables off the skewers on to a plate. Pour over the peanut sauce and serve.

## SPICY TOMATO SOYA FILLETS

Preparation time: 30 minutes
Cooking time: 35 minutes
Serves 2

4 plain soya fillets
400ml passata (sieved tomatoes, available from
    supermarkets)
4 tablespoons extra-virgin olive oil
2 cloves garlic, crushed
5 mushrooms, finely chopped
8 cherry tomatoes
3 tablespoons red wine
1 tablespoon pine nuts
1 red chilli, deseeded and chopped (optional)

Preheat the oven to 180°C/350°F/Gas Mark 4. To make
the marinade, mix together the passata, olive oil, garlic,
mushrooms, chilli, fructose, red wine and tomatoes. Place
the fillets in a shallow ovenproof dish, and pour the
marinade over. Cover and marinate in the fridge for half
an hour. Toast the pine nuts in a dry pan for 4 minutes,
until golden, then add to the marinade. Cover the dish
with baking foil and cook for 20 minutes. Remove the foil
and cook for a further 15 minutes.

## AVOCADO AND FETA SALAD

Preparation time: 10 minutes
Serves 1–2

3 very ripe tomatoes, skinned and diced
2 very ripe avocados, skinned and diced
125g plain feta cheese, cubed
3 tablespoons Greek yoghurt
juice of 1 lemon
25g chopped fresh coriander

Mix all the ingredients together and serve with baby salad
leaves, cucumber and onion.

## PENNE WITH MUSHROOM PESTO AND ASPARAGUS

Preparation time: 30 minutes
Cooking time: 10 minutes
Serves 6

1.5kg asparagus
480g penne pasta
30g butter or olive-oil-based spread
Parmesan cheese and toasted pine nuts, to garnish

For the mushroom pesto:
4 tablespoons extra-virgin olive oil
175g fresh mushrooms, sliced
20g dried porcini mushrooms, soaked for 10 minutes in a
   cup of hot water
1 tablespoon garlic, chopped
50g pine kernels
50g Parmesan cheese, grated
4 tablespoon fresh parsley, chopped
freshly ground black pepper

Heat the olive oil in a large pan over a medium heat, add
the fresh mushrooms and sauté. Drain and chop the
porcini mushrooms, then add them to the pan along with
the garlic. Cook for 2 minutes, then place them in a food
processor. Add the remaining pesto ingredients and purée.
Season to taste.

Break the fibrous ends off the asparagus and discard. Cut
the stalks so that each piece is a little larger than the
penne, then cook in a large pan of water. When the
asparagus is just cooked, take it out of the pan (but keep

the water) and put it into a bowl of cold water. Drain, refresh under a cold tap and leave to drain. Add the penne to the asparagus water, bring to the boil and cook until al dente, then drain. Return the pasta and asparagus to the pan and stir in the butter or olive oil spread. Serve topped with the mushroom pesto, and decorated with shavings of Parmesan and a sprinkling of toasted pine nuts.

## BROCCOLI AND TOFU SALAD

Preparation time: 10 minutes
Cooking time: 10 minutes
Serves 4

285g firm tofu, cubed
300g washed and ready-to-cook broccoli florets
350g washed and ready-to-cook cauliflower florets
1 avocado
2 tablespoons fresh or bottled lemon juice
25g pecan nuts, coarsely chopped
25g walnuts, coarsely chopped
8 cherry tomatoes, halved
2 teaspoons wholegrain mustard
50ml extra-virgin olive oil

Cook the broccoli and cauliflower in boiling water until
tender. Drain and refresh under cold running water. Halve
the avocado, de-stone, peel, cube and place in a bowl with
1 tablespoon of lemon juice. Toss lightly. Put the avocado,
broccoli, cauliflower, pecans, walnuts and tomatoes in a
shallow dish and mix together. Place the tofu cubes on
top. Stir together the remaining lemon juice, mustard and
olive oil to make a dressing, then pour this on top of the
salad to serve.

# GREEN VEGETABLE MEDLEY

Preparation time: 10 minutes
Cooking time: 25 minutes
Serves 4

220g can chopped tomatoes, made up to 450ml
    with water
6 sticks celery, cut into 1cm slices
300g fine green beans, trimmed and halved, or 300g
    baby sprouts
1 vegetable stock cube
freshly ground black pepper
baby new potatoes, to serve

Place the tomato and water mixture in a saucepan,
crumble in the stock and add the slices of celery. Bring to
the boil, then reduce the heat, cover and simmer for 10
minutes. Add the fine green beans or baby sprouts and
simmer, covered, for a further 15 minutes. Season to taste
with black pepper. Serve with a few baby new potatoes.

## VEGETARIAN MEXICAN CHILLI

Preparation time: 10 minutes
Cooking time: 30 minutes
Serves 2

1 large onion, chopped
1 red pepper, chopped
1 medium courgette, chopped
1 can chopped tomatoes
handful closed-cup mushrooms, sliced
½ can kidney beans, drained
½ can pinto beans, drained
1 tablespoon olive oil
1 vegetable stock cube
paprika, cumin and chilli powder (quantity depending on
    desired heat)
freshly ground black pepper

Fry the onion in olive oil for 5 minutes and add a few
pinches of paprika, cumin and chilli powder. Add the red
pepper and courgette, and fry for a further 3 minutes. In a
large saucepan, empty the can of chopped tomatoes, along
with the mushrooms, stock cube, kidney and pinto beans.
Transfer the contents of the frying pan to the saucepan,
bring the mixture to the boil and simmer. Add pepper and
the desired amount of spice, then continue to simmer for
15–20 minutes, stirring regularly.

## ASPARAGUS CREAM PASTA

Preparation time: 10 minutes
Cooking time: 15 minutes
Serves 2

160g fresh pasta
225g asparagus, blanched and chopped
30g butter or olive-oil-based spread
3 spring onions, chopped
30g fresh chives, chopped
150ml cream or crème fraîche
2 teaspoons grain mustard

In a medium saucepan, boil the pasta for 3 minutes until cooked al dente. Melt the butter or olive-oil-based spread in a medium frying pan before adding the spring onions and chives, followed by the cream/crème fraîche. Turn up the heat to reduce the sauce. When the sauce has reduced, add the mustard and blanched asparagus. Remove the sauce from the heat. Drain the pasta and combine it with the asparagus cream sauce before serving.

## SPICY SWEET POTATO AND CHICKPEA STEW

Preparation time: 20 minutes
Cooking time: 25 minutes
Serves 4

250g cooked chickpeas
500g sweet potatoes, washed and sliced
2 red onions, peeled and sliced
3 cloves garlic, peeled and crushed
450g tinned chopped tomatoes
2 tablespoons extra-virgin olive oil
290ml water
2 teaspoons ground cumin
2 teaspoons ground coriander
1 teaspoon turmeric
1 fresh green chilli, deseeded and finely chopped
1 inch (2.5cm) piece ginger root, peeled and finely
    chopped (or 1 teaspoon ground ginger)
1 tablespoon grain mustard
1 lemon, grated zest and juice
2 tablespoons chopped fresh coriander
freshly ground black pepper

Heat the oil and gently fry the onions, potato and garlic
for 2–3 minutes. Stir in all the spices and cook for a further
2 minutes. Stir in the tomatoes, water and chickpeas, and
season well. Bring to the boil and simmer until the
potatoes are tender. If the mixture becomes too dry, add
some more water. Stir in the lemon juice and zest, and
fresh coriander.

## ROAST VEGETABLE TORTE
Preparation time: 20 minutes
Cooking time: 45 minutes
Serves 2

1 red, 1 yellow and 1 green pepper, seeded and cubed
2 medium courgettes, cubed
1 medium aubergine, cubed
200g tinned or fresh artichoke hearts, drained and halved
1 large onion, peeled and sliced
225g ricotta cheese
4 free-range eggs, beaten
5 tablespoons extra-virgin olive oil
4 bay leaves
2 sprigs rosemary
2 sprigs oregano
3 teaspoons mixed Italian herbs

Preheat the oven to 200°C/400°F/Gas Mark 6. Place the vegetables and fresh herbs into a roasting tray and cover with the olive oil. Bake for 10–15 minutes. Combine the roast vegetables with the cheese, eggs and herbs. Pack the mixture into a 25cm flan dish and bake for 30 minutes.

## LEEK AND STILTON QUICHE (CRUSTLESS)

Preparation time: 20 minutes
Cooking time: 55 minutes
Serves 4

500g leeks, sliced
100g Stilton cheese, cubed
2 tablespoons extra-virgin olive oil
25g butter or olive-oil-based spread
350g onions, finely sliced
2 garlic cloves, crushed or finely chopped
3 eggs
275ml double cream/crème fraîche
1 tablespoon ground almonds
2 tablespoons freshly grated Parmesan
freshly ground black pepper
mixed salad, to serve

Heat the oil and butter or olive-oil-based spread in a pan until melted. Add the garlic, leeks and onions, and cook until golden brown and soft. Allow to cool slightly. Fold in the almonds and seasoning. Beat the eggs and cream together and add to the onion mix. Fold in the Stilton and half the Parmesan cheese. Spoon the mixture into a buttered flan case and sprinkle with the remaining Parmesan. Bake in a preheated oven (190°C/375°F/Gas Mark 5) for about 50 minutes until golden brown and set. Serve with a mixed salad.

# VEGETARIAN CURRY

Preparation time: 10 minutes
Cooking time: 30 minutes
Serves 2

8 new potatoes, chopped
3 tablespoons extra-virgin olive oil
knob of butter (optional)
1 small onion, chopped
400g tin chopped tomatoes
400g tin chickpeas, drained
1 tablespoon curry powder of your choice
freshly ground black pepper
green salad, to serve

Cook the potatoes in a medium pan until medium-soft. Drain the water and add the olive oil (and knob of butter, if desired). Add the onion, curry powder and black pepper (according to taste). Mix thoroughly. Add the can of tomatoes and chickpeas. If the mixture is very thick, add some water. Put the lid on the pan and braise the curry for 10–15 minutes. Serve with a green salad.

## PEA AND MINT FRITTATA

Preparation time: 10 minutes
Cooking time: 5 minutes
Serves 1

100g fresh peas, shelled
¼ bunch fresh mint, chopped roughly (reserve a few leaves
   for garnishing)
1 teaspoon young pecorino cheese, grated (Parmesan,
   Manchego or even a medium Cheddar would be fine)
50g Parmesan, grated
1 lemon
3 free-range eggs
1–2 tablespoons extra-virgin olive oil
50g butter or olive-oil-based spread
1–2 tablespoons crème fraîche
freshly ground black pepper
mixed salad, to serve

Preheat the oven to 180°C/350°F/Gas Mark 4. Quickly
plunge the peas into boiling water to soften or, if small and
sweet, just wash. Place in a mortar with the mint and grated
pecorino, and mash them to a paste. Add a little Parmesan
cheese, a squeeze of lemon juice and the olive oil. Melt the
butter or spread in a non-stick, ovenproof frying pan. Break
the eggs into a bowl, mix lightly, add a splash of water and
season. Add the mixture to the pan and then fold in the pea
mix, stirring once or twice. Place the crème fraîche in the
middle and bake in the oven for 3 minutes. Slide on to a
plate and serve sprinkled with the reserved mint leaves and
the remaining Parmesan. Serve with a mixed salad.

# PASTA WITH COURGETTES AND CREAM CHEESE

Preparation time: 10 minutes
Cooking time: 10 minutes
Serves 2

160g pasta
1 tablespoon extra-virgin olive oil
6 courgettes, diced
150ml cream cheese, whipped until smooth
1 lemon, half thinly sliced and half juiced
2 shallots, finely chopped
2 cloves garlic, crushed
1 red chilli, finely chopped
handful parsley, roughly chopped
freshly ground black pepper
1 tablespoon grated Parmesan, to garnish
handful torn basil leaves, to garnish

Boil the pasta until cooked al dente. Sauté the shallots, garlic and chilli in the olive oil and add the lemon slices. Next, add the courgettes and a little more oil if necessary, and fry until golden brown. Add the chopped parsley, cream cheese and lemon juice. Stir until the cheese has melted into the mixture to make a sauce. Season with pepper. Toss with the pasta and serve scattered with Parmesan and basil leaves.

## VEGETARIAN SAUSAGES WITH ROASTED VEGETABLES AND SWEET TOMATO SAUCE

Preparation time: 10 minutes
Cooking time: 20 minutes
Serves 1

4 vegetarian sausages
1 tablespoon extra-virgin olive oil
1 courgette, peeled and cut into long strips
1 onion, peeled and cut into 8 wedges
freshly ground black pepper

For the sauce:
400g can chopped tomatoes
1 tablespoon tomato purée
1 garlic clove, peeled and chopped
1 teaspoon dried chilli flakes, crushed
2 tablespoon balsamic vinegar
1 tablespoon red wine
1 teaspoon fructose

Scatter the courgette and onion on to a roasting tray. Drizzle with oil, season and roast in the oven for 10–12 minutes. Heat some oil in a pan and fry the sausages as per the packet instructions. To make the sauce, pour the tomatoes into a saucepan over a medium heat. Stir in the remaining ingredients and bring to the boil. Reduce the heat and simmer until reduced by one third. Slice the sausages in half on the diagonal. Serve the sausages and roasted vegetables topped with tomato sauce.

# GREEK SALAD

Preparation time: 10 minutes

Serves 1

100g feta cheese, cubed
1 large tomato, deseeded and chopped
½ red onion, peeled and chopped
50g drained pitted black olives
1 tablespoon chopped fresh flat-leaf parsley
baby new potatoes, to serve

For the dressing:
3 tablespoons extra-virgin olive oil
½ lemon, juice only
freshly ground black pepper

Whisk together the dressing ingredients in a small bowl.
Mix together the salad ingredients in a large bowl. Pour
the dressing over the salad and serve with a few baby
new potatoes.

# SOUFFLÉ OMELETTE WITH FRESH HERBS AND CHEESE

Preparation time: 10 minutes
Cooking time: 5 minutes
Serves 1

3 large eggs, separated
1 tablespoon single cream/crème fraîche
2 tablespoons each of parsley, dill and tarragon, chopped
salt and freshly ground black pepper
25g butter or olive-oil-based spread
drop of olive oil
55g grated Cheddar or soft goat's cheese
green salad, to serve

Put the egg yolks, cream, herbs and salt and pepper into a bowl, and mix. Whisk the egg whites until stiff, then take a large metal spoon and add 1 tablespoon of the egg whites to the yolk mixture, to slacken it a little. Then fold in the remaining egg whites. In a large omelette pan, melt the butter spread and the oil. Pour in the egg mix and cook on a medium heat. Do not stir or move but, when just beginning to set, sprinkle with the cheese. Flip one half over and cook for a further minute until cooked through. Serve with a green salad.

## CHEESE AND CHIVE MUSHROOMS

Preparation time: 10 minutes
Cooking time: 30 minutes
Serves 1


4 large open mushrooms
100g cream cheese
1 teaspoon reamed garlic
1 teaspoon chopped chives
50g fresh breadcrumbs (use Burgen bread)
25g Parmesan, grated
1 teaspoon chopped fresh parsley
freshly ground black pepper
extra-virgin olive oil, to drizzle

Preheat the oven to 180°C/350°F/Gas Mark 4. Cut the stalks off the mushrooms and lay them in an ovenproof dish, underside up. Mix together the cream cheese, garlic and chives, and season. Divide the mix into four and spread over the mushrooms. Then mix the breadcrumbs with the parsley and Parmesan, and season. Cover the top of the mushrooms with the crumb mixture and drizzle lightly with the olive oil. Bake in the oven for 30 minutes until the top is golden.

# DRESSINGS AND DIPS

## Dressings

To make these delicious dressings, simply shake all the
ingredients together in a jam jar or a bottle, or whiz them
with a hand blender.

### DIJON DRESSING
30ml balsamic vinegar
1 clove garlic, finely chopped (or ½ teaspoon garlic
   powder)
1 teaspoon Dijon mustard
1 teaspoon lemon juice
120ml extra-virgin olive oil
freshly ground black pepper

### BALSAMIC AND FRESH LEMON DRESSING
30ml balsamic vinegar
2 teaspoons fresh lemon juice
120ml extra-virgin olive oil
freshly ground black pepper

### CAESAR SALAD DRESSING
60ml white wine vinegar
90ml extra-virgin olive oil
4 teaspoons grated Parmesan
2 anchovy fillets, chopped
2 cloves garlic, chopped (or 1 teaspoon garlic powder)
freshly ground black pepper

## HOT AND SPICY DRESSING

30ml extra-virgin olive oil
120ml white wine vinegar
1 clove garlic, chopped (or ½ teaspoon garlic powder)
½ teaspoon mustard (any type)
pinch cayenne pepper

## CREAMY DRESSING

30ml extra-virgin olive oil
60ml cider vinegar
120ml plain yoghurt
½ teaspoon Dijon mustard
½ teaspoon basil
¼ teaspoon tarragon
freshly ground black pepper

## Dips

HOUMOUS

175g can chickpeas
3 tablespoons tahini paste
3 cloves garlic
3 tablespoons lemon juice
2 tablespoons extra-virgin olive oil
handful chopped parsley
pinch paprika

Put the chickpeas, tahini paste, garlic (you can use less or more as you wish) and the lemon juice in the blender. As it blends, add approximately 2 tablespoons of olive oil in a slow trickle. Taste the dip and, if it appears too 'dry', slowly drizzle in more oil. Put into a serving bowl and sprinkle with a pinch of paprika. Serve with crudités or salad.

## TUNA DIP

1 tin tuna
1 small onion, finely chopped (or chopped chives)
1 tablespoon olive oil
1 teaspoon grain mustard
lemon juice
parsley or coriander, chopped, to garnish

Drain the tuna. Mix together the mustard, lemon and olive oil. Then, using a fork, mash the tuna, the lemon and oil mix and the chopped onion together. Garnish with parsley or coriander. Serve as a dip with fresh crudités.

## SMOKED MACKEREL PÂTÉ OR DIP

1 packet smoked mackerel (the one with cracked pepper for extra zing)
1 tub cream cheese – for a pâté
1 tub Greek-style yoghurt – for a dip

Remove the skin from the mackerel fillets, then break up the fillets into a bowl. Carefully remove all bones. To make a pâté, mash the mackerel with the cream cheese until well combined. To make a softer dip, mash the mackerel with the yoghurt. Put into bowls and serve with crudités.

## RED SALMON DIP

1 large tin red salmon
2 tablespoons low-fat mayonnaise
¼–½ teaspoon chilli powder
½ cucumber, sliced and halved
juice of ½ lemon

Drain the salmon and mix it with the lemon juice, mayonnaise and chilli powder. Then add the cucumber and serve with crudités.

## TZATZIKI

1 tub Greek-style yoghurt
1 clove garlic, crushed
½ cucumber
handful fresh mint (3 teaspoons dried mint, if no
    fresh available)

Peel the cucumber and chop into small pieces, then crush the garlic and chop the mint finely. Put all in a mixing bowl with the yoghurt. Mix well, transfer to a serving bowl and serve chilled with crudités or as a side dish for meat dishes.

## DESSERTS

If you feel like a dessert, the best option is always low-GL fruit (see the list on page 40. However, the following recipes have been adapted to lower the overall GL by switching high-GL ingredients with lower ones – in other words, replacing sugar with smaller amounts of fructose, white flour with ground almonds, and normal chocolate with the dark chocolate that has a higher cocoa content.

Some of the recipes are quite high in fat and calories, so exercise caution. Still, it's good to know you can have these desserts when you fancy a treat, or for a special occasion, without ruining your good intentions!

### QUICK CHOCOLATE SPONGE PUDDING
Preparation time: 5 minutes
Cooking time: 3 or 15 minutes
Serves 2

2 free-range eggs
1 tablespoon cocoa
100g ground almonds
1 teaspoon baking powder
3 teaspoon fructose
25g melted butter or olive-oil-based spread
sugar-free cream or crème fraîche, to serve

Whisk together the melted butter or olive-oil based spread and eggs. Then add the dry ingredients and whisk thoroughly. Place in a microwave-proof pudding bowl and cook in the microwave on high for 3 minutes, or until springy on top. If you prefer not to use a microwave, you can bake the mixture in a greased muffin/cake tin in the oven for approximately 15 minutes, or until springy on top. Serve with fresh cream (sugar-free 'squirty' cream) or crème fraîche. For a special occasion you could serve with a tablespoon of vanilla ice cream!

'I lost 2 stone (13kg), dropped two dress sizes and changed my overall shape with the Diet Freedom GL Diet, and I have maintained the loss, despite introducing more moderate- glycaemic foods. I found the change of eating habits very easy. Instead of a saunter, I can now walk briskly. Having read a lot of books on the GI, I think the overall GL is the crucial part.'

*Brenda C, Lincoln*

## VARIOUS MUFFINS

Use the same recipe for Quick Chocolate Sponge Pudding on page 159 to make the following individual muffins:

Strawberry muffins
    remove the cocoa and add a handful of chopped
    strawberries to the mixture.
Apple and cinnamon muffins
    remove the cocoa and add a chopped apple and a
    teaspoon of cinnamon to the mixture.
Orange/lemon muffins
    remove the cocoa and add two teaspoons of orange or
    lemon oil (available from supermarkets).
Chocolate chunk muffins
    add small pieces of 70% cocoa chocolate to the mixture.

Either bake in the oven in a non-stick muffin tin for around 15 minutes, or bake individually in the microwave using small ramekins (about 1 minute each). Be very careful not to overcook the mix – it is ready when light and springy on top.

## STRAWBERRY AND FRESH FIG BRÛLÉE
Preparation time: 15 minutes
Serves 4

125g ripe fresh figs, sliced
125g fresh strawberries, halved
150ml double cream
150ml crème fraîche
1 vanilla pod (or 1 teaspoon vanilla essence)
4 egg yolks
2 teaspoons fructose
1 teaspoon fructose for sprinkling

Place the fruit into and around the edges of 4 large ramekin dishes. Place the vanilla pod in a pan. Stir in the two creams and heat to just below boiling point. Remove the pod. Beat the egg yolks and fructose together in a pan, then gradually beat in the hot vanilla cream. Heat gently until the sauce has thickened. Pour the custard over the fruit in the ramekins and set aside to cool. When cool, chill for 2–3 hours until set. Sprinkle the puddings with a little fructose and grill under a preheated hot grill to form a caramelised coating. Serve cold.

*Variations: you can change the fruits to any low-GL ones if you prefer, or use frozen fruits such as summer fruits or raspberries.*

## QUICK STRAWBERRY ICE CREAM
Preparation time: 5 minutes
Serves 2

1 small punnet strawberries, frozen
2 tablespoon single cream

Place the frozen strawberries in a blender and add the cream until an ice-cream consistency forms. Serve immediately.

## BLUEBERRY AND APPLE CRUMBLE
Preparation time: 10 minutes
Cooking time: 10 minutes
Serves 2

2 dessert apples, peeled, cored and sliced
handful blueberries
2 tablespoons water
25g porridge oats
2 teaspoons extra-virgin olive oil
1 dessertspoon fructose
2 tablespoon Greek yoghurt

Put the apples in a small pan with the water, cover and
cook gently until the apples have softened. Stir in half of
the blueberries and remove from the heat. Allow to cool.
Meanwhile put the oats, oil and fructose in a frying pan
and cook, stirring constantly until the oats are golden.
Allow to cool. Divide the apple mixture between two
dessert glasses and spoon the oat mixture on top. Top each
dessert with a tablespoon of Greek yoghurt and remaining
blueberries.

# GRILLED PEARS WITH RASPBERRY CREAM
Preparation time: 10 minutes
Cooking time: 4 minutes
Serves 1

1 pear, halved
1 teaspoon fructose
2 tablespoons Greek yoghurt
handful raspberries (reserving a few to serve)

Scoop the cores from the pear halves and place the fruit, cut side up, in a flameproof dish. Dust with the fructose and cook under a preheated moderate grill for 3–4 minutes until beginning to colour. Put the yoghurt into a small bowl, fold in the raspberries, then spoon the mixture into the centre of each pear half. Serve decorated with a few raspberries.

## PAN-COOKED APPLE CRUMBLE

Preparation time: 15 minutes
Cooking time: 30 minutes
Serves 4


5 apples
125g ground almonds
2 tablespoons grated lemon rind
100g chilled butter or olive-oil-based spread
40g fructose


In a large bowl, mix together the ground almonds and
lemon rind. Cut 50g of the butter spread into pieces and
use your fingertips to rub it into the mixture until coarse
crumbs are formed. Stir in the fructose, then put the
mixture in the freezer for 20 minutes. Meanwhile, peel,
core and chop the apples. Melt the remaining
butter/spread in a pan, add the apples and cook, stirring
constantly, for 10 minutes. Then cover and cook for a
further 5–10 minutes until tender. Transfer the apples into
an ovenproof dish and move to a warm oven. Wipe the
pan clean, add the crumble and cook over a medium heat
for 5 minutes, without stirring, until golden. Spoon the
apples into 4 bowls and top with crumble.

## STRAWBERRY AND MELON SALAD
Preparation time: 10 minutes

225g small strawberries
1 small melon
1 firm kiwi (over-ripe fruit have a higher GL)
squeeze of lemon juice
2 tablespoons freshly squeezed orange juice (or juice
     with bits)
plain/Greek yoghurt or crème fraîche, to serve

Wash and hull the strawberries. Peel and slice the kiwi. Slice the top of the melon, carefully making a zigzag pattern with the knife. Then remove the seeds and scoop out the flesh with a melon-baller or a teaspoon. Keep the shell to one side. Mix all the fruit together in a bowl and stir in the lemon and orange juices. Transfer the fruit salad to the melon shell and serve with plain/Greek yoghurt or crème fraîche.

CHOCOLATE TORTE

(for special occasions – a healthier celebration cake!)

Preparation time: 10 minutes

Cooking time 1 hour

Serves 4

50g almonds

50g walnuts, shelled

150g dark chocolate, 70% or 85% cocoa solids (such as
   Lindt or similar)

½ teaspoon cocoa powder

125g butter or olive-oil-based spread

40g fructose

3 large free-range eggs, separated

cream or crème fraîche, to serve

Preheat the oven to 190°C/375°F/Gas Mark 5. Line an 8
inch cake tin with greaseproof paper, and grease the
bottom and sides. Grind the nuts in a food processor until
finely ground. Then add the chocolate and cocoa powder,
and grind for 30 seconds to break up the chocolate. Put
into a mixing bowl and set aside. Place the butter/spread
and fructose in the food processor and beat until pale and
fluffy. Add the egg yolks one at a time, then fold this
mixture into the chocolate and nut mixture. In a separate
bowl, beat the egg whites until stiff peaks form, then fold
into the chocolate mixture. Pour the mixture into the
cake tin and bake for approximately 25 minutes, or until
springy on top. Serve with cream or crème fraîche.

*Chocolate with added nuts generally means a lower overall GL.*

# RASPBERRY BRÛLÉE

Preparation time: 10 minutes
Cooking time: 5 minutes
Serves 4

175g fresh or frozen raspberries
400ml double cream
200ml crème fraîche
1 vanilla pod
5 egg yolks
30g fructose
two teaspoons fructose for sprinkling

In a saucepan, heat the creams with the vanilla pod to just below boiling. Remove from the heat and take out the vanilla pod. Whisk the egg yolks and fructose in a bowl until light and slightly thickened, then add to the warm creams. Place the saucepan back on the heat and stir until custard coats the back of the spoon. Divide the raspberries equally between 4 ramekins and pour over the custard. Chill for 2–4 hours in the refrigerator. When cold, sprinkle ½ teaspoon of fructose over each ramekin, then carefully place them under a preheated hot grill. Heat until the fructose forms a crispy topping. Allow to cool before serving.

## ALMOND FARM CAKES

Preparation time: 5 minutes
Cooking time: 20–30 minutes
Makes 12 cakes

50g fructose
2 egg whites
½ teaspoon vanilla essence
125g ground almonds

Preheat the oven to 150°C/300°F/Gas Mark 2. Mix the fructose into the egg whites and whisk slightly until the fructose is well incorporated. Add the vanilla essence and ground almonds. Transfer the mix to a piping bag and pipe small rounds on to greaseproof paper. Place a split almond on top of each farm cake. Bake for 20–30 minutes or until golden brown. Leave to cool before removing from the baking tray.

*Variations: Add a dessertspoon of cocoa powder for a chocolate version!*

# RED WINE AND CINNAMON POACHED PEARS

Preparation time: 10 minutes
Cooking time: 10 minutes
Serves 2

2 large pears
½ bottle red wine
1 teaspoon fructose
1 cinnamon stick
½ tub soft cheese
cream, crème fraîche or Greek yoghurt, to serve

To prepare the pears, peel and cut off the base so they stand upright. Boil the red wine, adding the fructose and cinnamon. Then add the pear and poach until soft. Remove and chill. When cold, cut off the top of the pear and remove the core. Fill the gap with the cream cheese before replacing the top. Serve with crème fraîche, cream or Greek yoghurt.

# BAKED LEMON AND VANILLA CHEESECAKE

Preparation time: 20 minutes
Cooking time: 30 minutes
Serves 6

200g cream cheese
200g ricotta cheese
juice and rind of 1 lemon
1 vanilla pod
120g fructose
4 eggs, separated
150ml double cream/crème fraîche
low-GL fruit slices or raspberry/strawberry purée, to serve

Grease an 8 inch loose-bottomed cake tin. In a large bowl, mix together the cheeses, lemon juice and rind, seeds from the vanilla pod, fructose, egg yolks and double cream. Whisk the egg whites until firm, using an electric hand whisk. Gently fold the egg whites into the cheese mixture and pour into the cake tin. Bake at 170°C/325°F/Gas Mark 3 for approximately 30 minutes. Turn off the oven, open the door and allow the cheesecake to cool in the oven. Serve decorated with low-GL fruit slices or a raspberry/strawberry purée.

## LEMONY SPONGE CAKE

Preparation time: 10 minutes
Cooking time: 40 minutes
Serves 4

100g olive-oil-based spread or butter
100g fructose
175g ground almonds
1 teaspoon baking powder
2 medium free-range eggs
4 tablespoons milk
finely grated rind of 1 lemon

Preheat the oven to 180°C/350°F/Gas Mark 4. Grease and line a 8 inch (20cm) cake tin with non-stick baking parchment. Put all the ingredients into a large bowl and beat well for 2 minutes until smooth. Turn the mixture into the tin and level the surface. Bake in a preheated oven for about 35–40 minutes, or until the cake has shrunk slightly from the sides of the tin and springs back when lightly pressed. Leave in the tin until cold, then turn out and remove the paper.

## WILD BERRIES WITH FROZEN YOGHURT
Preparation time: 20 minutes
Freezing time: variable
Serves 4

150g frozen summer fruits
350g plain yoghurt
100ml single cream/crème fraîche
75g fructose
100g strawberries
100g blueberries
100g raspberries
100g blackberries
(or whatever combinations of fresh berries are available)

Place only the frozen fruits in a small pan and heat gently, stirring until thawed. Transfer them to a food processor and blend until smooth. Chill until ready to serve. Stir together the yoghurt, cream and fructose, and place in an ice-cream maker. Churn for 20–25 minutes, or until the mixture has frozen. If you don't have an ice-cream maker, pour the mixture into a shallow container, place in the freezer for 1 hour, then transfer to a food processor and blend until smooth. Freeze for 2 hours, and then process again before freezing until firm. Hull and quarter the strawberries and place in a bowl with the blackberries, blueberries and raspberries. Stir in the puréed sauce and divide between 4 bowls. Spoon the frozen yoghurt on top.

# 7

# The Low-GL Shopping Guide

Let's be practical for a moment ... in an ideal world it would be great if we could all grow our own food, cook everything we eat from scratch and never open a packet again! But for most of us that's merely a pipe dream. We have to go food shopping and ready meals and convenience food are features of modern life.

So, we've put together the definitive low-GL shopping guide ... Or how best to get out of the supermarket without a basket full of temptingly marketed, fattening junk foods!

First, try to eat before you shop. Being hungry normally equates to overflowing baskets/trolleys filled with quick-fix, high-GL foods! These glucose fixes are all too easy to consume on the way back home in the car ... Second, skip the aisles full of the highly processed foods that made you put on weight, and that you don't eat any more – such as biscuits, cakes, pastries, sweets, and so on.

So how do you normally shop? Are you a list-maker or do your cravings do the shopping?

As you first start the GL Diet, you may find it easier to make a list and stick to it. However, once you have the GL

Diet habit, you'll have the confidence to be more of a 'spur of the moment' shopper.

Before you shop, you may find it helpful to sit down with this book and plan how your fridge, freezer and cupboards need to be restocked. Think:

- fresh (where possible)
- natural ingredients
- low hassle
- low GL

Here are a few ideas …

## FRIDGE

- Semi-skimmed milk/unsweetened soya milk
- Small pot of single cream or crème fraiche
- Unsweetened 'squirty' cream
- Cheese – half-fat cheese is a very good choice, but you do get a lot of taste from a relatively small amount of the stronger cheeses such as Stilton and Parmesan
- Olive-oil-based spreads
- Bio yoghurt/low-fat, Greek-style yoghurt

## FRESH FRUIT AND VEGETABLES

Choose from the low-GL food lists (Chapter 4), bearing in mind that fresh food won't last too long. Grapes, grapefruit, pears, plums, strawberries, or whatever you fancy – try to buy smaller quantities, more often, so it stays fresh. Apples and tangerines are a great convenient snack to have in the house. And don't forget lemons (and limes): they give a great zing to so many foods and dressings. They've also been shown to lower the overall GL of meals.

## BAKERY
Choose low-GL breads such as Burgen or pumpernickel.

## STORE CUPBOARD
- Any other beans and pulses from the food lists
- Butter beans (tinned if easier – look for no-added-sugar version)
- Chickpeas (tinned if easier – look for no-added-sugar versions)
- Couscous
- Desiccated coconut (unsweetened)
- Dried apricots
- Extra-virgin olive oil
- Ground almonds (to take the place of flour in baking)
- Herbs and spices. All herbs and spices are truly secret weapons. Foods can be so much tastier with a few fresh herbs, or experimental blend of spices, and you don't need any added salt
- Nut oils such as walnut or macadamia
- Pesto
- Reduced-sugar baked beans
- Seeds – linseeds, pumpkin seeds, sunflower seeds, sesame seeds
- Sundried tomatoes in olive oil
- Tinned fish (tuna, sardines, and so on)
- Tinned tomatoes (no added sugar)
- Traditional oats (steel-cut oats preferably)
- Unsalted nuts – almonds, hazelnuts, macadamia nuts, walnuts, pecans, pine nuts, peanuts
- Unsweetened bran sticks (available from health-food shops)

- Vinegar – balsamic, red and white wine vinegar or flavoured vinegars

## MEAT AND FISH COUNTER

All meats and fish have a low GL. Choose lean meats that are as natural as possible without too many additives. Try to balance the amount of red meat and white meat you buy, and be sure to remember lots of fish!

## FREEZER SECTION

There are a lot of temptations to be found here. However, there are also lots of good foods that can make cooking quick and easy.

Frozen vegetables are a great standby and they retain all their nutritional quality, as they are usually frozen quickly after picking/harvesting. These days there's an ever-increasing choice, from broad beans, cabbage, carrots, green beans, leeks, peas, spinach, sprouts, sweetcorn, or mixed vegetables … Choose your own favourites from the low-GL vegetables list in Chapter 4.

Frozen fruit is also very handy. Store summer fruits, such as blueberries, raspberries and strawberries, and blend for a cool summer smoothie – or try some of the dessert recipes using frozen fruits (see page 169, Chapter 6).

Frozen fish, chicken and other meats in their natural state are all low GL. Natural is always best – skip or minimise the breaded and battered processed products. Frozen prawns are quick to defrost and make delicious stir-fries and curries. They're also great for salads and prawn cocktails.

## HEALTHY, 'FAST' MEALS FOR WHEN
## YOU ARE IN A HURRY

We all have days when we need to get home and eat something that takes five minutes to cook. No preparation – just five minutes in the microwave and hey presto! There's no doubt that some pre-prepared supermarket meals have ingredient lists that read like the contents of a chemical laboratory. But increasingly you can find healthy pre-packaged meals, or at least the basis of a meal, that includes quality food, with little in the way of additives and preservatives.

Always glance at the label. The shorter the lists of ingredients (the less tampered with) the better. If you understand what they all are, and they sound like basic food items – great!

It's possible to get lots of variation in fish or meat dishes with sauces. Avoid anything with rice, pasta or potatoes. Also look to see if there is sugar, glucose or high-fructose corn syrup added and whether it features high on the list of ingredients – the higher it is, the greater its content. Ideally there should be no added sweetener.

The following sauces all provide good accompaniments to beef, chicken, pork or fish: cheese, Madeira, mushroom, tomato, tomato and basil, spinach and ricotta, tomato and mascarpone, red pepper, black pepper, white wine, red wine, tarragon, forestière, pesto, watercress, chasseur, asparagus, spinach and nutmeg.

Some of these ready-made meals will be quite high in fat, but the 'light' options normally contain a lot more sugar and additives, so beware!

Avoid sweet and sour or barbecue sauces because they

are loaded with sugar – as are Chinese meals with sauces. Indian chicken- or prawn-based meals with sauces, such as balti, jalfrezi, madras, korma or tikka masala, are all fine. And it is now becoming increasingly popular to eat these meals with salads instead of rice, which is a great idea and surprisingly delicious!

Sadly, the pre-packed vegetarian options are mainly pasta- or rice-based, but you can sometimes find tofu- or Quorn-based meals.

If you need some 'fast' vegetables to stick in the microwave, there are plenty to choose from – cauliflower cheese, green vegetable selections, bags of mixed vegetables, Mediterranean vegetable medleys.

There are lots of lovely ready-made salad combos too – ones with salad, egg and a few slices of new potato are great, or any that are colourful and look appetising. By combining one of the main dishes listed above with fast vegetables or a salad, you have a relatively healthy and speedy, low-GL meal – far better than grabbing a burger and chips or a pizza.

## FAST DESSERTS

The best options are fresh fruit, pre-packed fruit salads, melon medleys (normally with no added sugar) or sugar-free yoghurt. Sadly most pre-packed desserts have one thing in common: they are loaded with sugar (often listed as the first ingredient!). So avoid chemical-laden double-toffee or triple-chocolate concoctions with a high GL. Choose a delicious fresh fruit salad or dive into a melon medley – savour the fresh taste and *enjoy* feeling virtuous!

'Four years ago, while working as a police officer, I had a very bad car accident and I haven't been able to exercise since. The only way I have been able to keep my weight down is by following a low-glycaemic diet. I am very interested in health and nutrition and the Diet Freedom GL Diet approach makes perfect sense to me. I have found the GI books confusing and contradictory but using the GL, which takes into account the actual portions and the carbs within them, is far better and more accurate. Using the GL, instead of the GI alone, I can now have a greater variety of foods, which makes it less restrictive and easier to stick to. I tried Atkins a year ago but lasted a week, as I found it terribly boring.

*Stephen B, Notts*

# 8

# The Low-GL Eating-out Guide

## BEFORE YOU GO

Most of us don't eat out all the time, so let's enjoy ourselves when we do by making the best selections we can and eating delicious food.

Have a long drink before you go – preferably water (often we confuse hunger with thirst). It will make you feel fuller so you eat less.

Have a piece of cheese or a piece of fruit to help take the edge off your appetite. Don't skip meals earlier in the day as an excuse for a 'blow out' later – it doesn't work!

Try to put yourself in the right frame of mind before you arrive at the restaurant. Why are you going out? What is the focus of the evening/party/event? Ninety-nine per cent of the time, it won't be the food, it will be the people, the celebration, the event itself. Focus on the people and enjoying the party. Picture yourself looking as you want to look, feeling confident and happy. Picture your plate, the foods on it, the delicious healthy choices. Picture yourself feeling pleasantly full, smiling as you graciously refuse seconds or a high-GL food. Picture yourself coming home, having had a great time, and feeling happy that you've enjoyed the evening so much.

## PARTY TIME

When it comes to social gatherings and parties, try to find out what the food choices are likely to be. Dropping subtle hints to friends that you are reducing bread, pasta, potatoes, rice and sugar in your diet as they don't suit you (if you don't want to say you are losing weight) is normally all it takes. For birthdays, weddings and other celebrations, venue managers are perfectly used to special requests for vegetarians, coeliacs and various other dietary requirements, so don't be shy to ask for what you want.

If pasta, pizza, potatoes or rice form the basis of a main course, put the bare minimum on your plate and load up on vegetables, salad or the fish/meat available – the GL of your meal will then stay low to moderate.

## BUFFET CHOICES

Most likely we will all be confronted with a plate, a napkin and a laden buffet table at some point, so what are the best low-GL choices from popular buffet-style foods?

Savouries:
- All meat and fish (except for anything breaded or battered)
- All salads
- Eggs/curried eggs/egg mayonnaise (except Scotch eggs)
- Quiche (pastry is high GL – eat the middle and leave the rest)

- Sausage rolls (eat the sausage and leave the roll)
- Caesar salad
- Coleslaw
- Avocado salad/dips
- Tomato salad
- Cheeses
- Prawn cocktail
- Smoked salmon
- New potatoes (three or four are OK)
- Potato salad (a small portion if you aren't having any other potatoes)
- Olive-oil-based dressings

Most dips are fine if their base is yoghurt, mayonnaise or tomato.

Skip the following: pasta salad, rice salad, sandwiches and rolls (avoid, if possible, or choose the darkest, grainiest bread and discard the top piece), garlic bread, sugar-filled desserts.

## DESSERTS
- Fruit
- Fruit salad
- Cheese with grapes and celery – no biscuits

*If there are only sugar-filled high-GL desserts on offer, ask the waiting staff for fruit or cheese instead.*

## RESTAURANTS – WHAT SHALL I HAVE?
We have such an incredible choice of places to eat these days, so here are a few general guidelines, followed

by advice on what to order when eating a certain kind of cuisine.

- If the vast majority of the food on your plate is low GL, you can get away with adding small portions of moderate- to high-GL foods. The overall GL will still be fairly low – so no need to feel deprived!

- Feel confident in telling the waiter/waitress that you cannot eat foods or sauces high in sugar/flour and ask them to check that the food you have ordered doesn't contain those ingredients. Food intolerances are extremely common, so waiting staff are perfectly used to such requests.

- When you sit at the table, explain that you don't want any bread – it saves the temptation of a hovering breadbasket!

- Thankfully, many pubs and restaurants are now taking notice of their customers' increasing health awareness and are adapting their menus to suit. At Diet Freedom we are campaigning hard for GL labelling! Across the board, one of the best low-GL choices is lean meat or fish and vegetables or salad.

- Pepper is a great condiment and gives the food a better zing than salt – you really don't need to add extra salt to your food.

- If you aren't sure about the sauces, ask for a plain tomato or cheese sauce. Ask if your fish/meat dish could be served with a different sauce from the menu, or ask for no sauce but extra vegetables and salad.

- Ask the waiting staff what vegetables are on offer – reject the potatoes/French fries and order double of the low-GL vegetables instead.

- If you can't see any main courses you like the look of, why not have two starters – generally the starters menu will have a bigger choice of lower-glycaemic options. For example, prawn cocktail/salad is ideal – even though the sauce will be slightly sweetened, it's not enough to worry about. And most vegetable soups, without potato or rice added, are low GL and extremely filling. Other great starters are avocado and prawns, melon, feta or goat's cheese, scallops ... There are numerous tasty options.

- When choosing desserts, avoid high-sugar pastries and puddings. Instead ask for cheese with grapes, celery or apple (no biscuits). Even if they are not listed on the menu, most restaurants will oblige. Good choices are a fresh fruit salad, a piece of fruit, a bowl of strawberries or melon with cream/sugar-free yoghurt. A small amount of ice cream (no wafers) is the next best option. The plainer the better – chocolate, strawberry or vanilla. Despite containing sugar, it's relatively low GL.

## ITALIAN

Pasta and pizza normally spring to mind when 'Italian food' is mentioned, the latter being one of the highest-GL foods on the planet. However, there are lots of delicious low-GL ways to eat Italian-style:

- Ignore the pasta and pizza dishes. The GL of pasta is higher the longer it has been cooked and some restaurants will reheat it, cooking it twice, so it is best avoided when eating out. Most Italian restaurants do have a wide selection of alternatives with interesting and tasty fish, meat and vegetarian options.

- Good olive oil, balsamic vinegar and Italian dressings are always available, and make delicious salads with freshly grated Parmesan.

There are many wonderful low-GL starters to choose from:

- Tuna Niçoise salad – a perfect low-GL dish with added olives and anchovies.
- Tricolore Salad (Insalata tricolore) – avocado, tomato and mozzarella salad, usually with fresh basil and dressing.
- Carpaccio – thinly sliced raw beef, often served with crisp salad, horseradish and shaved Parmesan. Sometimes you will also see Tuna Carpaccio, which is prepared the same way but with tuna instead of beef.
- Antipasto – a selection of assorted meats and cheeses.
- Seafood salads, grilled calamari, frittata, pesto, prawns.

## MEXICAN

- Stick to just one tortilla (preferably flour rather than corn).
- Good food choices include: grilled fish or meats, chicken wings, guacamole and salads. Big salads are regular fare in Mexican restaurants and usually include cheese, chilli con carne, guacamole, salsa, and so on – very filling. If the salad comes in a giant taco, ask if it can come in a bowl instead!
- Try to avoid: quesadillas, nachos, tacos, chimichangas, burritos and enchiladas.

## GREEK

The flavours of good Greek cuisine are second to none. The wonderfully creative use of herbs and spices provides some fabulous dishes with a very low GL:

- Grilled fish, meats and vegetables are abundant on Greek menus.
- The salads are often a delicious combination of leaves and fresh herbs – usually dressed in olive oil and lemon juice or vinegar.
- Spiced sausages (loukanika) and cured meats are low GL but quite high in salt and fat, so keep them to a minimum.
- Chickpeas and pulses are very heavily used. All are low GL – so enjoy the aubergine dip, houmous or tzatziki.
- Bread will almost always be offered. Try to say no, but if you do choose to have it then a small piece of pitta bread is your best bet – as long as the GL of the rest of your meal is kept to a minimum.
- Kebabs – delicious grilled meat or vegetables, very tasty with the dips (without the bread).
- Fasolia Gigandes and Fasolada – butter bean stew and white bean soup.
- Aubergine – as a vegetable or a dip.
- Halloumi cheese.
- Horiatiki – a classic Greek salad of tomato, cucumber and olives.
- Stefado – a very tasty beef stew.
- Moussaka – this dish primarily consists of meat and aubergine, which is fine, but often contains potatoes and lots of fat, so have only small amounts and load up with salad.

## INDIAN

- All rice has a very high GL, so is best avoided. Why not try salad as an alternative accompaniment? The combination is surprisingly good.
- Also avoid: biryani (rice), naan bread, onion bhajis, pakoras and samosas. A chapatti would be a better option than naan if you can't resist something to mop up the sauce!
- Most dishes with traditional Indian sauces (such as those based on cream, onion, tomato, yoghurt and spices) will be low GL. Some sauces can be quite high in fat, so use your discretion. Many dishes are made to order, so be sure to ask for no sugar in your choices. Acceptable dishes include: Bhuna, Korma or Tikka Masala with meat, fish or seafood, plus any of the plainer meat and fish dishes. Raita is a delicious yoghurt-and-mint-based dip that is low GL – and cool to eat with the spicy Indian dishes!
- Indian cuisine is very inventive vegetable wise, using plenty of beans and pulses, okra and spinach, so it's good to fill up on those.

## CHINESE, JAPANESE, THAI

### Chinese

- The rice used in Oriental restaurants is normally the short-grain variety that has the highest GL of all. Also avoid the sweet and sour dishes and stick to some of the more delicious 'fresh' options, like the griddled meats, fish and vegetables. Most Chinese sauces will contain corn flour and sugar, but you can always ask for no sauce.

- Good choices: Crispy Duck, provided you skip the plum sauce and just have one small pancake if you can't resist. Get your chopsticks clicking and tuck into the duck, cucumber and spring onion! Also: beef with Chinese mushrooms, prawn platter, chicken with walnuts, chicken with sweetcorn, chicken with cashew nuts, or similar pork dishes.
- MSG or monosodium glutamate is a flavour enhancer that is often added to Chinese foods – it overexcites the taste buds on your tongue and can lead you to overeat! In the shops MSG is sometimes listed directly on food labels but it is more frequently hidden in other ingredients, such as yeast extract, autolysed vegetable protein, or hydrolysed vegetable protein – so beware!

## Japanese and Thai

Thai food has many excellent low-GL dishes based on coconut milk and meat or fish, while Japanese food is considered to be very healthy and, aside from the sticky rice, this is generally the case. The curries are great, and even tempura (fish, shellfish or vegetables, fried in light batter) will be fine. Choose sashimi over sushi. Sashimi is thinly sliced, raw seafood that is chilled and eaten with wasabi (Japanese horseradish mustard) and soy sauce. Sushi also uses raw fish, but rice is the base of most sushi dishes.

## FAST FOOD

Of course, most of it will be high GL! But there are ways around it. Here are a few ideas:

- Swap the hamburger with the bun for a hamburger

with salad. Or, better still, don't bother with the burger at all!

- Swap the breaded deep-fried chicken and fish (unhealthy trans fats) for non-breaded if available.
- French fries have a whopping GL of 50 for 150g – just say NO! Apart from the unhealthy trans fats, they will make you store fat.
- Have an 'open' sandwich (discard the top bit of bread). Then you can actually see what you are eating!

Not all 'fast food' is bad. Many sandwich shops and fast-food outlets are now offering healthier options:

- The sandwich chain Prêt à Manger now has the 'breadless sandwich' alongside its other delicious salads.
- Benjys sandwich chain is very diet aware and provides an interesting range of snacks.
- Some of the larger fast-food chains are now incorporating salads into their menus.
- And if you simply must have Full English Breakfast, or fry-up, every once in a while, stick with the eggs, bacon, tomatoes, sausage and mushrooms and you'll be fine.

## COFFEE SHOPS

Coffee chains often add sugar syrups to their drinks, so make sure you ask for a plain coffee with either milk, pouring cream or whipped cream.

## SNACKS

So easy, so quick – so often very high GL!

- Crisps – potato crisps have a moderate to high GL so

are best avoided. Celeriac crisps are a better alternative and they taste surprisingly good.

- Nuts are extremely calorie dense, so watch the amount you consume (no more than a handful a day), but they are a very low-GL option. Particular heroes in the nut world are heart-healthy almonds and Brazil nuts (high in selenium, a powerful antioxidant) but all nuts are generally healthy and nutritious.

- Seeds – linseeds, pumpkin seeds and sunflower seeds are all great low-GL choices, with many added health benefits. Pumpkin seeds and sunflower seeds also make fabulous snacks. Look for the tasty mixed-seed bags in health-food stores and some supermarkets.

- Both nuts and seeds are also naturally high in fibre – another big tick in the box.

- Chocolate – joy of joys, some chocolate is fine! Cocoa is actually very good for you. However, many chocolate bars include a huge amount of sugar and saturated fat and precious little cocoa. The high-cocoa chocolate options (look for at least 70% cocoa solids) such as Lindt or Green & Black's are perfectly acceptable – a few squares now and then won't provide too much sugar or set off cravings. Also they have a rich taste, so you are less likely to overindulge.

- Cereal/snack bars – generally not a good choice. Even the natural ones, sold as health bars, are often very high in some form of sugar – sadly brown sugars and organic sugars have the same effect on blood sugars as white table sugar. Beware of the low-carb and diabetic chocolates available – they can have serious (and sometimes immediate) laxative effects! They contain the controversial polyols (or sugar alcohols), such as maltitol, some of which have been tested to be very high glycaemic. It is claimed that they are not digested as normal carbs and therefore they are excluded from the 'net' carb count on the label. This is very misleading to customers, as low 'net' carbs doesn't necessarily equal low GI/GL. This is probably why low-carb dieters often complain that they stall their weight loss! The laxative effects sadly DO NOT contribute to losing fat, by the way!

## ALCOHOL

Most of us like a drink every now and then. However, while you are shedding those unwanted pounds you will shed them faster without alcohol. It doesn't help that the more we drink the lower our willpower becomes, where food is concerned. A case of one thing leading to another! So if you do fancy a tipple, choose red wine over white, dry white wine over sweet, slimline tonic or diet mixers with spirits, and try to keep your consumption moderate! Reduced-carb lagers, such as Michelob Ultra, are now available from most supermarkets.

## DRINKS IN GENERAL

Stick with coffees with no sugar or added syrups, teas, herbal teas, bottled waters, sugar-free smoothies, soya milk, sugar-free soya smoothies, tomato juice, vegetable juices such as V8 or home-prepared vegetable and fruit juices, sugar-free cordials and diet drinks with no added sugar.

'I wanted to lose 12 lb (5kg) and, although other diets had worked, it was the beginning of a new year and I felt like a new "challenge"! Sometimes a fresh approach is what you need to kick-start you. Not only did the Diet Freedom GL Diet plan work, I reached my target weight in two months and found my digestive problems virtually disappeared – no more bloating, and so on. But what I really appreciate is the food education I got. The more I know about food, and its effect on me, the more able I am to make sensible, balanced choices about what I eat without becoming a pernickety food-faddist.'

*Margaret S, Warwickshire*

# 9

# Love Your Food, Love Your Body

Good things we can do for our health:
- Drink plenty of water
- Eat good food
- Get active
- Laugh a lot

Most of us know about the basics of healthy eating. However, it can sometimes seem daunting trying to make sure we're eating enough of the things that are 'good' for us and not too much of the things that are 'bad'. Often we just give up and leave it to chance.

At last you can relax. GL Diet recipes and food lists take care of all of that for you. So you can get on with your life, as well as look and feel great, and still enjoy fabulous food, with the comfort of knowing you are getting all the good nutrition you need.

Sometimes understanding some of the science and a few of the facts behind healthy-eating messages can make it that bit easier to see why we should all be making some changes, so this chapter looks at some of the main points and explains them in plain, simple language.

## WHAT'S SO GOOD ABOUT FRUIT
## AND VEGETABLES?

Apart from the fact that most fruit and vegetables are great for low-GL eating, what makes them so important are antioxidant vitamins and minerals.

Antioxidants are the good guys. They roam around the body mopping up 'free radicals' and basically sacrifice themselves to save the cells in our bodies. Free radicals, the bad guys, are deformed or incomplete compounds that we pick up from a variety of sources: pollution (over 70,000 chemicals are pumped into the air every day!), stress and smoking, to name but a few. The only way the bad guys can survive is to attach themselves to our cells, but this eventually damages or kills our cells, and leads to more free radicals and a vicious circle for our health.

Fruit and vegetables are loaded with antioxidants, and the more we eat the more protection we have from free-radical damage, heart disease and some cancers. There are lots of different kinds of antioxidants, such as vitamins A, C and E – the ACE vitamins – as well as minerals like selenium. To make sure you're getting enough, you need to eat a minimum of five portions of different-coloured fruit and vegetables every day.

Taking a good-quality multivitamin and mineral supplement can be a good insurance policy to support a healthy diet, but it can never replace all the benefits of eating real nutrients from real foods.

## WHAT'S CLASSED AS A PORTION?

A portion of fruit is:

- 1 medium-sized piece of fresh fruit – for example, half a large grapefruit, a slice of melon or 2 satsumas;
- 2–3 small pieces of fruit (plums or apricots);
- 1 handful of grapes;
- 7 strawberries;
- 3 heaped tablespoons of fruit (stewed or tinned in juice);
- 1 small glass (150ml) of unsweetened fruit juice;
- 3 dried apricots.

A portion of vegetables is:
- 3 heaped tablespoons of cooked vegetables (carrots, peas or sweetcorn);
- 1 side salad (the size of a cereal bowl);
- 1 tomato or 7 cherry tomatoes.

## THE BOTTOM LINE

Eating at least *five* portions of different-coloured vegetables and fruit a day is our first line of defence against free-radical damage and disease, and a potent form of preventative medicine.

## SALT – THE FACTS

Ninety per cent of us eat too much salt – and many of us eat as much as double the recommended safe levels. Just imagine if 90% of us drank double the recommended amount of alcohol every day, or 90% thought it was OK to smoke – and, even worse, if we thought it was acceptable for our children to do the same!

In the past, concern about salt intake has focused mainly on the middle-aged with high blood pressure and heart trouble, but all of us are eating far too much salt, and the consequences for our health could be dramatic.

On average we are eating 10–12g of salt a day, whereas the recommended maximum intake for an adult is 5–6g or one flat teaspoonful. Too much salt increases the risk of blood pressure, a major cause of strokes and heart attacks in the UK. High salt intake may also be associated with osteoporosis, fluid retention, asthma and stomach cancer.

The problem is that so much of the salt in our diets is hidden in processed foods. Often salt isn't listed on food labels and it gives the sodium content instead. To make sense of sodium on food labels, multiply the sodium amount by 2.5 – that tells you how much salt is actually in the product.

---

Practical recommendations to lower salt intake:
1. Whenever possible, make your own meals from scratch and leave out the salt.
2. Don't use salt at the table.
3. Reduce the amount of salt in cooking by trying alternative seasonings such as black pepper, herbs, spices, lime and lemon juice.

---

## GOOD FATS, BAD FATS?

The most recent research strongly advocates using olive oil and avoiding hydrogenated or trans fats, which are highly processed and have been linked with cancer and heart disease. Some researchers and nutritionists now recommend olive oil or small amounts of butter instead of the low-fat margarines and spreads, which often contain trans fats or hydrogenated oils. Many highly processed foods, such as biscuits, cakes, cereals and chocolate bars, also contain hydrogenated fats, although there are now recommendations to reduce or ban them completely.

Studies have shown that people who use the most olive oil are significantly less likely to develop rheumatoid arthritis and may also reduce their risk of developing colon cancer. Adding olive oil to the diet has other advantages as well. The cardiovascular benefits of diets higher in olive oil are well established in improving the ratio of good to bad cholesterol.

These findings may help to explain the heart-healthy benefits of the Mediterranean diet, which is rich in olive oil, fruits and vegetables. (Try to remember that not ALL cholesterol is bad – LDL is the baddie and HDL is the 'good' cholesterol. LDL takes cholesterol to the arteries and HDL takes it away from the arteries, back to the liver for disposal.)

All these benefits could be achieved by including olive oil in our daily diet. Use it in cooking and make up your own dressings. Your GL Diet recipes include several delicious olive-oil-based dressings. Usual shop-bought dressings often have added sugar and salt, so make your own whenever possible – that way you know exactly what is in it and it only takes a minute! If you have less than a minute, a simple squeeze of fresh lemon juice and a splash of extra-virgin olive oil will put a zing into any salad combination.

There are now several olive-oil-based spreads available in the supermarkets, including supermarket own-brand spreads. They taste good, contain no or very low levels of unhealthy hydrogenated fats, and are also lower in saturated fats. This makes them great for all types of cooking and baking, and a good alternative if you prefer not to use butter.

## THE BENEFITS OF OMEGA-3
## FOUND IN FISH OIL

Omega 3 helps fight and prevent heart disease and has also been linked to reducing the risk of cancer, depression, Alzheimer's, arthritis, diabetes, ulcers, hyperactivity and many other diseases.

While a helpful form of Omega-3 can be found in flaxseed and walnuts, the most beneficial form of Omega-3 containing the two essential fatty acids DHA and EPA can only be found in fish oil.

A lot of people take cod liver oil. It is a very popular supplement that most people know about. However, you need to ensure it is from a reputable source, because if it is a by-product of the in-shore fishing industry it can contain pollutants called 'dioxins'. The bottom line is you get what you pay for. Of course the best option is just to eat more fish like salmon, trout, mackerel, sardines and herrings, as well as plenty of white fish (we've recently discovered hoki, which is delicious).

## WATER

Most of us know we don't drink enough water, and it can seem daunting to hit the target of 1.5–2 litres a day.

Water is essential for life. Each of us is made up of around 60% water. The nutrients from our food are transported around the body by water and most of the chemical reactions that go on in the body need water. All of these reactions produce waste products and, yes, you've guessed it, without water we couldn't get rid of any of that waste.

Just like a car radiator, water flows through the body to help maintain the right temperature. We constantly lose water in our breath and through sweat and, if we don't replace the lost water, we're in danger of overheating!

What happens if I don't drink enough? A lot of people don't even realise they are dehydrated, because they have become so used to feeling below their best. Dehydration can leave you feeling tired, constipated, nauseous and can often result in frequent headaches.

## How do I know if I'm dehydrated?

A good way of knowing if you are drinking enough is by the colour of your urine! If it's pale and straw-coloured, you're OK; any darker and you would probably benefit from drinking more.

## So, how much do I need?

In a moderate climate like the UK, most of us need around 6–8 cups or glasses of water each day to keep the balance right. In hotter climates this amount increases. Likewise, if we take part in strenuous exercise, we need more water than usual to help us keep cool. A good guide is 1 litre of extra water for every hour of strenuous exercise.

## But what if I don't like drinking water?

Some people do find water unpalatable but you can make it more interesting by adding slices of lemon and lime.

Diluted unsweetened fruit juice is also a good way of jazzing water up if you find it boring. Fruit and herb teas also make good hot drinks which will help you keep hydrated.

## Does tea and coffee count?

Drinks like tea and coffee and some fizzy drinks contain caffeine, which is a diuretic and can cause further fluid losses. However, drinking caffeinated drinks is better than not drinking at all. If you do drink lots of tea, coffee or cola, try swapping every other drink for water. Start gently and build up your water intake every few days.

## Do I have to drink special water?

If you prefer bottled or filtered water that's fine. There are those who say tap water is OK to drink straight from the tap and those who say it is dangerous and the added fluoride is also a health hazard. Tap water has to have chemicals added to make it safe and kill all the nasties. As to what effect these chemicals have on us, the jury is still out – so you'll need to make your own decision there.

The overall message is: water is vital to our survival, so drink plenty!

'I was due to have a hip-replacement operation and needed to lose weight but was told that, as I was in constant pain, could barely walk with a stick and certainly couldn't do any kind of exercise, this would be virtually impossible. Because of the pain the temptation to comfort eat was also a problem. I decided to go along (with my stick!) to the Diet Freedom meetings at my local health club – and lost 11 pounds (5kg), which is a lot for me as I am only 4 ft 10 (1.5m)! I found the educational side and relearning what to eat an inspiration. The weight loss gave me a real psychological boost and I have now had both my hips replaced and am recovering well. I have also recommended the Diet Freedom GL Diet to many of my friends who are also losing weight. The recipes are quick and easy – just as well, as my husband has been doing the cooking while I have been ill!'

*Jane R, North Cockerington, Lincs*

# What Do Doctors and Scientists Say About GL?

'Although the GI of a food is helpful information, it is only part of the story, because the effect of eating a food on blood glucose and insulin levels depends on both the amount of carbohydrate and the GI of that carbohydrate. For this reason the concept of the **"Glycaemic Load" or GL** has been developed. This is the amount of carbohydrate in a food multiplied by the Glycaemic Index of that carbohydrate. The GL better reflects a food's effect on your body's biochemistry than either the amount of carbohydrate or the GI alone. This is important – some diet books have warned against eating carrots because they have a high GI, which slanders this fine food that only has a small amount of carbohydrate.'

Walter C Willett MD Dr PH, Chairman of the Department of Nutrition at the Harvard School of Public Health and Professor of Medicine at Harvard Medical School.

'As an advocate of low-glycaemic eating for everyone, especially those suffering from chronic illness, I'm delighted that at last a book has appeared that takes this concept to the next level. Its beauty is in the simplicity and logic of its ideas, allowing people to eat not only low-glycaemic foods but to mix them with higher-glycaemic foods to enable them to enjoy a much more satisfying and varied diet. Why didn't anyone think of it before! It's certainly a book I will be making available in my clinic as part of my patients' treatment plan. The route to the restoration and maintenance of good health starts with nutrition, and the concept of Glycaemic Load or GL will help me best advise my patients how to eat in the future.'

Dr Andrew J Wright MBChB DRCOG MRCGP DCH DIHom
runs the Complete Fatigue Clinic in Bolton, Greater Manchester.
A GP and specialist in integrated medicine.


## THE RESEARCH

Researchers at the Harvard School of Public Health, based in Boston, USA, have carried out the longest and largest studies into health and diet in the world. They are now recommending a low-glycaemic diet and producing guidelines based on it.

Clinical studies have shown that low-glycaemic foods and drinks are beneficial to humans: 'Clinical use of Glycaemic Index as a qualitative guide to food selection would seem prudent in view of the preponderance of evidence suggesting benefit and absence of adverse effects.'

The Journal of the American Medical Association (JAMA),
8 May, 2002

'Studies from the Harvard School of Public Health indicate that the risks of diseases such as type II diabetes and coronary heart disease are strongly related to the GI of the overall diet. In 1999, the World Health Organisation (WHO) and Food and Agriculture Organisation (FAO) recommended that people in industrialised countries base their diets on low-GI foods in order to prevent the most common diseases of affluence, such as coronary heart disease, diabetes and obesity.'

Professor Jennie Brand Miller, University of Sydney, 2004

'Pregnant women who eat sugary or highly processed foods, known as high Glycaemic Index foods, may have an increased risk of neural tube defects such as spina bifida, in their newborns. The risk doubled for women who ate a lot of these foods, and among obese women the risk quadrupled.'

*The American Journal of Clinical Nutrition*, November 2003

'Researchers have found that people who eat "low-quality carbohydrates" have high blood levels of C-reactive protein (CRP), a powerful promoter of inflammation. The finding is significant because growing research indicates that inflammation of blood vessels is at the root of heart disease and many other common degenerative diseases. High CRP levels increase the risk of heart attack by 4.5 times. Women who consumed large amounts of potatoes (mostly mashed and baked), breakfast cereals, white bread, muffins, and white rice had the highest CRP levels.

It is conceivable that high glycaemic foods may also stimulate the inflammation characteristic of arthritis, asthma, and many other diseases.'

*The American Journal of Clinical Nutrition*, 2002, 75:492–498

'Research into dietary fibre, Glycaemic Load and diabetes risk in women revealed that the dietary Glycaemic Index, as well as the dietary Glycaemic Load, was positively associated with risk of diabetes. The more high glycaemic carbohydrates consumed, the greater the incidence of diabetes. Fibre intake was associated with a decreased risk of diabetes. Researchers concluded that diets with high Glycaemic Load and low fibre intake increase risk of diabetes in women. Further, they suggest that by consuming minimal amounts of refined carbohydrates, the incidence of diabetes can be reduced.'

*The Journal of the American Medical Association*, 277(6), 1997

'When dietary Glycaemic Load was assessed by a food frequency questionnaire in postmenopausal women the results revealed that as Glycaemic Index, carbohydrate intake and Glycaemic Load increased, levels of HDL ("good") cholesterol decreased and triglycerides [triglycerides are another fat found in the blood which, at high levels, are detrimental to heart health] increased. The relationship between Glycaemic Load and elevated triglycerides was greater in women who were overweight. Researchers concluded that this study supports the physiologic relevance of the Glycaemic Load as a potential risk factor for coronary artery disease in women, particularly those prone to insulin resistance.'

The American Journal of Clinical Nutrition, 73(3), 2001

'Diets high in refined starches such as breads and cereals increase insulin levels. This affects the development of the eyeball, making it abnormally long and causing short-sightedness, suggests a team led by Loren Cordain, an evolutionary biologist at Colorado State University in Fort Collins. Over the last 200–250 years the average Glycaemic Load of foods in urban areas of industrialised countries has risen steadily, primarily because of increasing consumption of refined cereals and sugars. This increase in sugars is clearly related to increased levels of insulin.'

Acta Ophthalmologica Scandinavica, March 2002

'Dietary Glycaemic Load has been significantly associated with an increased risk of colorectal cancer. Researchers speculate that a diet prominent in foods with high glycaemic indices, like white bread and white rice, affect insulin factors or exacerbate inflammatory responses and, thereby, increase the cancer risk.'

Women's Health Study in the Journal of the National Cancer Institute, February 2004

'We speculate that the prolonged satiety associated with low GI foods may prove an effective method for reducing caloric intake and achieving long-term weight control.'

*Pediatrics*, 111(3), 2003

A study published in *Pediatrics* (112(5):e414) in November of last year found that children eating a low-GI breakfast tended to eat more moderately throughout the day, while those eating a high-GI breakfast were more likely to be hungry by lunchtime.

Top US dermatologist to the stars and best-selling author of *The Wrinkle Cure* Dr Nicholas Perricone bases his work on a simple premise: aging skin and other dermatological conditions are the result of inflammation at cellular level. He recommends a low-glycaemic diet for healthy, youthful skin and also to treat acne. Sugary foods and highly refined carbs can cause inflammation in the skin leading to wrinkles.

US researchers fed diets made up of 69% carbohydrates to two groups of rats. However, one group of 11 rats was given high-GI carbohydrates and 10 were given low-GI carbohydrates. After 18 weeks they found the high-GI group had 71% more body fat and 8% less lean body mass than the low-GI group. They also had higher levels of triglyceride blood fats, another heart disease risk factor in humans. The rats also showed the sort of changes linked in humans to a high risk of diabetes. In a further experiment, 24 mice were randomly assigned a low- or high-GI diet. After nine weeks, the high-GI group had 93% more body fat than mice on the low-GI diet.

Dr David Ludwig, who led the team at the Children's Hospital in Boston, USA, commented, 'What the study shows is that Glycaemic Index is an independent factor that can have dramatic effects on the major chronic diseases plaguing developed nations – obesity, diabetes and heart disease. The Atkins diet tries to get rid of all carbohydrates, which we think is excessively restrictive. You don't have to go to this extreme if you pay attention to the Glycaemic Index and choose low-GI carbs.'

Lancet 2004; 364:778–85; DB Pawlak, JA Kushner, DS Ludwig DS. 'Effects of dietary Glycaemic Index on adiposity, glucose homoestasis and plasma lipids in animals'

'In type II diabetics, a low glycaemic diet significantly lowers fasting serum fructosamine and cholesterol levels after only two weeks.'

TM Wolever, DJ Jenkins et al. Department of Nutritional Sciences, Faculty of Medicine, University of Toronto, Canada

'A study of 42,759 male health professionals reported in *Diabetes Care* showed that a high Glycaemic Load increased the risk for men to get type II diabetes.'

*Diabetes Care*, April 1997; 20(4): 545–50

'I had been diagnosed with Polycystic Ovary Syndrome (PCOS), and had been trying to lose weight for years with very slow progress. I literally thought the only way I would ever get the weight I'd gained off was by starving myself. I couldn't believe it when I found the Diet Freedom GL Diet – food I loved, never feeling hungry and, best of all, I dropped two dress sizes in just over a month! The weight is easy to keep off, because Diet Freedom has just become a way of life. I have the energy and the enthusiasm to exercise and feel so positive – it's like I've been put back in the driving seat!'

*M McCall, Bucks*

# 11

# Your Questions
# Answered

### Is this a low-fat diet?
No, the GL Diet is based on healthy fats such as olive oil, with recommendations to avoid unhealthy hydrogenated fats and trans fats found in many processed foods, and to keep saturated fats to a minimum.

### Will I have to count calories?
No, by eating meals with a low GL you will not be promoting fat storage via blood-sugar highs and lows and, providing you stick to the few quantity limits for certain foods, there is no need to count calories. It has been suggested that you can eat approximately one-third more calories on a low-GL diet, while still losing weight, which means it is far more sustainable and you won't feel deprived.

### Are there any supportive products available for the GL Diet plan?
You do not need to buy ANY products at all to follow the Diet Freedom GL Diet plan, but for those of you who (like us) are short of time, we have painstakingly developed a range of natural, low-GL, GMO-free snack/convenience

products to keep you (and us) on the low-GL track when temptation strikes! So far we have a low-GL wrap, which is very tasty and versatile – in fact you can eat it on its own! We also have hand-baked celeriac crisps and a roasted, toasted seed mix.

## How will I know which foods have a low Glycaemic Load?

We have provided you with simple lists of low-GL foods, specially developed low-GL recipes and advice on how to choose healthier low-GL 'speedy meal' options. So you don't have to think 'What can I have that is low GL?' It's all been worked out for you!

## Can I eat desserts?

Yes, but they are optional. We provide dessert recipes and ideas for special occasions. If you need to have a dessert every day, stick to low-GL fruit or a sugar-free yoghurt.

## How quickly will I lose weight?

The GL Diet is a healthy diet based on sound nutrition and the latest research. It is NOT a quick-fix fad diet. We try to be honest and straightforward, so you won't find us promising you will lose a stone (6kg) in a week! Your weight loss will depend on many factors, including your age, exercise level, genes, general health, metabolism and the amount of weight you have to lose.

## Do I have to weigh myself regularly?

How you wish to keep track of your weight loss is your choice. We recognise that not everyone likes to get weighed, while others find it the only way to keep themselves on track. We do recommend using the Body Mass Index (BMI) chart as a guide towards a healthy weight based on your height.

The 'healthy' BMI range is 20–25. We recommend you decide on your ideal weight within that range as your target. If your BMI is over 30, aim for stepping stones of two points on the BMI scale at a time. Measuring is also an excellent way to gauge your progress, so you have the option to measure certain areas each week.

You will find a printable version of both the BMI chart and a measuring chart (with our advice on how to properly measure yourself) on our website www.dietfreedom.co.uk

### Can I drink alcohol?

Most alcohol is high in sugars and therefore high GL. You will lose weight far more easily if you choose to skip the alcohol. If you must indulge, though, wine is the best bet. Red wine has a lower GL than white, and research has shown that red wine does offer some health benefits. The sweeter the wine the higher the GL. Most spirits are OK in moderation. Generally the sweeter it tastes the higher the GL.

### Why do some people seem to eat all the wrong things and not put weight on?

We all know people who eat loads, including all the wrong things, and STILL never seem to put on any weight. They have been blessed with a genetically high metabolic rate, which means they will always be slim. The vast majority of us, sadly, have a slower metabolism and a genetic predisposition to store away fat. This means that, had we lived hundreds of years ago, we would have survived in times of drought and famine and our skinny counterparts would have perished! Now that food is (more than) plentiful, the ability to store fat to live off during future hard times is no longer the benefit it once was!

## Not losing weight? Could it be a thyroid problem?

This subject really is a book in itself, but in brief ...

Underactive thyroid problems (hypothyroidism) are extremely common and often mean people will find it 'extremely' difficult to lose weight. Many cases are not picked up as the symptoms are so diverse and can be attributable to many other causes.

One of the main symptoms is tiredness, sometimes accompanied by breathlessness. Dry skin and thinning hair are also common symptoms. A good description of having a failing thyroid is feeling like you are in 'hibernation' – only half functioning – no energy or zest or enthusiasm for life. The reason is that your thyroid, a bow shaped gland situated at the front of your neck regulates your metabolism. If it starts to fail, your metabolism slows down, your temperature falls and your body can't pump blood around your body fast enough to service all of your bodily functions, so as a safety mechanism it just concentrates on the most important organs to sustain life such as your heart and lungs. This is why two of the possible symptoms (and no two people will be the same) are dry skin and thinning hair. Because skin and hair aren't essential to sustain life they start to be affected adversely. Exercise will help, but telling someone to go out and exercise when they are hypothyroid and can barely keep their eyes open is not going to work!

If you think you may be experiencing some of the symptoms of an underactive thyroid, a good test to do at home is to check your temperature first thing in the morning on waking. Place the thermometer under your arm and leave it there for 10 minutes whilst relaxing. A normal temperature is 97.8–98.2°F. If your temperature is below this it may be an indication that your thyroid gland is struggling.

Your doctor may suggest a blood test to check your thyroid is working properly. This will include a TSH test, which tells you the level of 'thyroid stimulating hormone' in your blood. A raised TSH level is the first sign that your thyroid may be failing and means that your body is trying to stimulate itself to produce more thyroid hormone as you don't have enough to function properly. If your TSH level is above the normal range and you are exhibiting underactive thyroid symptoms your GP may prescribe a synthetic hormone called thyroxine, a small tablet which you have to take every day continuously to replace the missing hormone. This works extremely well for most people and it can mean that within a few months you will start feeling well again, have a lot more energy and actually feel like exercising.

If you are still struggling to lose weight despite following the guidelines in the book, it may be that you do not metabolise carbohydrates well – in which case we recommend you try the following:

- Eat plenty of vegetables, olive oil, pulses and fruit (to keep up your intake of fibre), and lean meats and fish

- Moderate your intake of bread, pasta, sugar and rice
- Moderate your intake of porridge/grain-based products
- To keep your calories in check also switch to lower-fat cheese, crème fraîche instead of cream, half-fat milk and avoid nuts

## Do I need to take a multivitamin and mineral supplement?

Whether you are on a diet or not, it is a good insurance policy to take a broad-based supplement each day. The foods we eat today are not as nutritious as they once were, due to depleted minerals in our soil and intensive farming methods. ALWAYS check with your GP before taking supplements, as some can interact with medications. If you don't like fruit, you may want to consider taking a good antioxidant.

## Is exercise part of the diet?

Exercise is vitally important, particularly if you are trying to lose weight. By taking regular exercise, you will improve your health and lose weight more quickly. Even three brisk 10-minute walks a day have been proven beneficial. Ensure that you check with your GP before embarking on a new exercise regime. Gyms and health clubs provide professionals to help you get started safely. Do something you enjoy and shake your body.

## What happens when I reach my target weight and size?

Well, first of all you don't want to lose any more weight, so introducing more food is the simple answer. However, if you return to your old eating habits, which made you put on weight in the first place, you will obviously start gaining.

By the time you have reached your desired size and shape you will not only see the benefits of eating a low-GL diet, but you will also feel far better health-wise, with increased energy levels, clearer skin and less irritating health problems such as colds, flu, sore throats, and so on. Another major benefit of balancing blood-sugar levels is increased emotional stability, with no sugar-induced mood swings and depression.

So, just stick with your low-GL principles and remember that eating low-GL foods is not just about losing weight but retaining and improving your health.

You may wish to have more regular low-GL desserts after your evening meal. If you haven't eaten nuts, a handful a day would be a good healthy addition. There is obviously room for a few treats here and there BUT do remember that, for some people, many highly refined high-GL foods such as a slice of white bread or sugar-filled chocolate may set off cravings and lead to binges.

Now you've got the low-GL habit, you will probably want to stick to the low-GL alternatives most of the time. You will soon gauge what you can eat and still maintain your new shape. Increase your food intake gradually and monitor the results.

If you haven't been doing any baking, try out some of the delicious low-GL dessert recipes. You can make lovely crumbles, muffins and sponge puddings using ground almonds and other white-flour substitutes, with small amounts of fructose instead of sugar to sweeten. You may also wish to increase your intake of bread when you would like to maintain your target weight. We recommend you use Burgen or pumpernickel bread.

And finally, there is one major problem with following the GL Diet that we feel we should warn you about (and your partners, come to think of it). You may well find it necessary to buy yourself a whole new wardrobe of clothes! But hey, life's tough!

### There is a lot of science involved; do I need to understand it?

No, the main criticism of the GI as a reference is that, because it is science based, it is difficult for the layperson to understand and doesn't translate very well into everyday use – which is why we wrote a book based on the GL rather than the GI. Glycaemic Load is a simpler and more accurate reference, which translates the science of the GI into a user-friendly eating plan. So all you need to do is follow the guidelines and food lists in this book. Simple!

### I want to know more about the science behind the GL Diet

You will find a lot more information on our website www.dietfreedom.co.uk where we constantly add new research and newly tested foods.

### Can I join a Diet Freedom club to follow the plan?

We have trialled the diet in a weekly club format with excellent results and have future plans to extend Diet Freedom clubs throughout the UK. In the meantime you can join fellow Diet Freedomers in our friendly online forums at www.dietfreedom.co.uk and 'buddy up' to others as a means of support. You can also use our 'ask the dietitian' advice.

> 'I have an underactive thyroid and take thyroxine so have always had a real problem losing weight. I have now lost over two stone with the Diet Freedom GL Diet and dropped two dress sizes. After trying every diet under the sun this is the only one that has worked and I have kept the weight off. I still have a stone to go but it is coming off steadily.'
>
> *Julia D, Grimsby*

We really hope you have enjoyed this book and that it has proved helpful.

If you require further information on the latest, up-to-date findings about how GL can help your health, or if you want to find out more about our low-GL food products please come and visit our website www.dietfreedom.co.uk or e-mail us at:
nigel@dietfreedom.co.uk
tina@dietfreedom.co.uk
deborah@dietfreedom.co.uk

( diet freedom )

# Recommended Reading

Brand-Miller, Professor Jennie: *The Glucose Revolution*: Marlowe and Company, 2004

Collier, Roz and Foster, Georgia: *Slim by Suggestion*: HarperCollins, 2001

Salmansohn, Karen: *How to Be Happy, Dammit: A Cynic's Guide to Spiritual Happiness*: Celestial Arts, 2001

Weil, Dr Andrew: *Eight Weeks to Optimum Health*: Time Warner, 1998

Willett MD, Walter C: *Eat, Drink, and Be Healthy*: Simon and Schuster, 2004